BRODART, CO.   Printed in U.S.A.

Hospice or Hemlock?

Hospice or Hemlock?

Searching for
Heroic Compassion

Constance E. Putnam

Foreword by Timothy E. Quill, M.D.

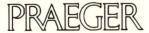

Westport, Connecticut
London

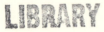
Library of Congress Cataloging-in-Publication Data

Putnam, Constance E., 1943–
    Hospice or hemlock? : searching for heroic compassion / Constance E. Putnam ;
foreword by Timothy E. Quill.
      p. cm.
    Includes index.
    ISBN 0–89789–921–0 (alk. paper)
    1. Hospice care. 2. Terminal care. 3. Terminally ill—Medical care. I. Title.
R726.8.P88 2002
361.1'756—dc21   2002070882

British Library Cataloguing in Publication Data is available.

Library of Congress Catalog Card Number: 2002070882
ISBN: 0–89789–921–0

First published in 2002

Praeger Publishers, 88 Post Road West, Westport, CT 06881
An imprint of Greenwood Publishing Group, Inc.
www.praeger.com

Printed in the United States of America

The paper used in this book complies with the
Permanent Paper Standard issued by the National
Information Standards Organization (Z39.48–1984).

10 9 8 7 6 5 4 3 2 1

Copyright Acknowledgments

The author and publisher gratefully acknowledge permission for use of the following
material:

John Stearns Hayward excerpt, from "When the wind blows . . ." in *Energy* (Ithaca, N.Y.:
[privately published], 1997), [n.p.].

Simon Dach, excerpt from "Wie ist es nicht gnug, einmal sterben lasser?" in Walter Ziesmer,
ed. *Gedichte*, 4 vols. (Tübingen, Germany: Max Niemeyer, GmbH, 1936), vol. 1, pp. 203–206.

for
Hugo
sine quo non

You have talked about this till you have come to be in love with—deposition and departure. But such is not the natural condition of a man.

—Anthony Trollope, *The Fixed Period: A Novel*,
edited by David Shelton, Oxford University Press, 1993, p. 36

I detest the doorways of death.

—Homer, *The Iliad*, University of Chicago Press, 1961, p. 206

Contents

Foreword *by Timothy E. Quill, M.D.*   ix

Preface and Ackowledgments   xiii

1. The Matter of Death   1

2. Origins of the Debate   25
   Starting with Hippocrates   28
   Hospice   30
   Profile: Dame Cicely Saunders   41
   Hemlock   44
   Profile: Derek Humphry   51

3. Whose Death Is It, Anyway?   65
   Kinds of Rights   69
   The Right to Die   70
   Killing vs. Letting Die   82
   The Integrity of the Profession   93

4. Dealing with Death   105
   Do-It-Yourself Help   110
   Profile: Jack Kevorkian   115
   Legal Help   118
   Profile: Herbert Cohen   129

Medical Help   132
Profile: Timothy Quill   135

5. Putting Principles into Practice   149
Using External Principles for Evaluation   149
Using Internal Principles for Evaluation   157
Pain and Dignity-of-Life Arguments   159
The Trajectory of a Life   161
Doctor-Patient Dialogue   164
Profile: Joanne Lynn   168

6. Death Matters   177
Common Ground, Compromises, and Conclusions   178
Consequences and Implications for Society   183
Heroic Compassion: Hospice and Hemlock   186

For Further Reading   197

Index   201

Foreword

In informal surveys of medical professionals as well as lay groups about their end-of-life wishes, I have consistently found little desire for either "hospice" or "hemlock." What colleagues, friends, and acquaintances all seem to want is to live as long as possible—as intact as possible—and then to die relatively quickly. Some prefer to die in their sleep, with no awareness or preparation, whereas others would prefer a short period (at most a week or two) of "death awareness" so they would have time to settle affairs and say "goodbye."

With the changing trajectory of dying in the developed Western world, probably fewer than 10 percent of us will die suddenly or after such a brief illness. Most of us will have a long period of chronic illness, perhaps punctuated with periodic acute exacerbations associated with slowly progressive decline in function, prior to our deaths. Furthermore, in part because medical technology is so effective at prolonging life, the end of this process will likely include hard choices about prolonging a diminishing life, or forgoing treatment with an implicit prior decision about accepting or even accelerating death. A "natural death," unencumbered by medical choices and interventions, is a rarity in our world.

It is in this context that the choice posed by Constance Putnam in her new book, *Hospice or Hemlock?: Searching for Heroic Compassion*, takes on a particular poignancy. The challenge she presents for us is how to respond compassionately to patients who are dying in the modern context (some of whom are suffering unacceptably after long periods of illness and decline), in particular those who want assistance in dying sooner rather than later. Much of the debate in the United States about how physicians should respond to requests for assistance in dying has focused on a forced choice between what she has characterized metaphorically as "hospice" and "hemlock."

Polarizing, "either-or" choices, debates, and rhetoric are peculiarly American. Superficial statements that overstate the positives of one's own position while casting the opposition in the worst possible light are elevated to an art form in media "sound bites." One must be either "pro-life" (opponents are "anti-life") or "pro-choice" (opponents are "anti-choice"), whereas the majority of those on both sides favor life and choice. Similarly, it sometimes seems we must choose between hospice—which "affirms life" and "relieves suffering"—on the one hand, and hemlock— which respects patient "self-determination" and "individual choice"—on the other hand. Not surprisingly, Putnam concludes that the majority of us want our lives to be affirmed and our suffering to be relieved *as well as* to have our individual choices and values listened to and respected at the end of our lives. The forced choice between compassion and self-determination ultimately turns out to be a false choice that serves no one particularly well.

Hospice as a philosophy of care focuses on aggressive management of pain and symptoms, so potentially dying patients can make the most out of the time that remains before life's end. There is an ideology to hospice that suggests a "good death" should not only have excellent symptom management, but also meaningful closure with one's family and peaceful acceptance of death as a natural end to the life cycle. For better, for worse, "good deaths" of this sort are not always achievable, nor are they even desirable in everyone's eyes. Putnam explores the historical, philosophical, and religious history of the hospice movement and writes critically about some of the hospice mantras such as "neither hasten nor postpone death" or "hospice respects patient choices and values." These statements sound good on the surface, but they tend to be misleading and sometimes fall apart on closer analysis. For example, hospice workers frequently and quite appropriately postpone death with the use of simple treatments such as antibiotics, in hopes of prolonging the life that a patient still finds meaningful. Conversely, death might be hastened at a patient's request provided that the method is indirect, such as stopping a potentially life-sustaining therapy (intravenous fluids, nasogastric tubes, steroids, or mechanical ventilators). Hospice's "respect for patient choices and values" is a qualified one, as the choices and values must be ones of which the program approves. If one is requesting the stoppage of a life support, then the message is to listen to the patient and respect his or her values. But if patients were to request physician-aid-in-dying by other methods (such as physician-assisted suicide or voluntary active euthanasia), then the message is a different one. Such patients must be depressed or confused, the thinking goes (if they were in their right mind, they would be satisfied with hospice care), or perhaps they are simply not getting enough hospice care. The notion that such patients might really know what they want or need is fundamentally called into question in most hospice contexts.

In Chapter 3, Putnam explores in considerable detail some of the philosophical and ethical distinctions that underlie the debate about what kind of assistance in dying is permissible, and what is impermissible. She begins by examining different potential implications of the "right to die" that individuals might have, and what kinds of duties might thereby be incumbent on physicians and others. She uses this analysis as background for a critical exploration of some of the cornerstone distinctions of modern ethical thinking about end-of-life decision-making, such as those between "killing" and "letting die," or between "active" and "passive" euthanasia, as well as the doctrine of double effect. Those on either side of the debate about the permissibility of physician-assisted death would do well to read her analysis, which pulls together information and ideas from a variety of scholars and fields, and addresses a large number of not easily answered questions.

Within hospice there has been a genuine struggle to respond to tough cases where unacceptable suffering occurs despite unrestrained efforts at palliation. The focus has mainly been on which methods of assistance are acceptable and which are unacceptable. Stopping or not starting a life support is acceptable even if the patient's intention is to die because we are "passively" assisting, and we are "allowing the patient to die of his underlying disease." Of course, if one stopped a life support against a patient's will, the defense that one was simply letting nature take its course would be preposterous. Thus we learn that there is something about the patients' values and consent, as well as their clinical circumstances, that is more fundamental than any distinction between active and passive assistance.

Furthermore, those who have argued that there is no need for physician-aid-in-dying because we can "relieve 100 percent of suffering" can only make this somewhat outrageous assertion by suggesting that we can resort to "terminal sedation" to allow an escape for the difficult cases. Terminal sedation involves sedating a patient to unconsciousness to permit escape from awareness of otherwise unrelievable suffering. (The physician's intent must be purely to relieve suffering, even though he can foresee that the patient will inevitably die, for the act to be protected by the doctrine of double effect.) Then food and fluids are withdrawn (withdrawal of life-sustaining therapy has wide legal and ethical acceptance). Some patients and physicians, when they look at the act in the aggregate, will see this as a self-deceptive form of "slow euthanasia," but for others these distinctions help maintain vital elements of the integrity of the profession. Even though terminal sedation is increasingly viewed as an acceptable alternative to other forms of physician-assisted dying by many in hospice and palliative care, its availability is very uneven, as is the acceptability of patients directly requesting such assistance if they experience or fear severe suffering.

Physician-aid-in-dying has been legally available in Oregon since 1997, so we are now beginning to get some empirical data to address questions about whether hospice and hemlock are really incompatible, or if they may complement one another. The data so far are very reassuring to those of us who believe that "hospice" should be the standard of care for the dying, but that "hemlock" should be openly and legally available as a last resort if suffering becomes unacceptable. First of all, there have been very few cases, and the majority of those patients who died under the Death with Dignity Law were simultaneously on hospice programs at the time they requested and received assistance. All patients met the legal criteria to be assisted under the law. Second, there were six requests for every potentially lethal prescription eventually written, suggesting a careful process of discrimination by patients and doctors. Third, there is ample evidence that hospice care has improved in Oregon since physician-aid-in-dying was legalized—morphine prescriptions per capita are up, more patients are dying at home, hospice referrals have increased, and more physicians are being trained in hospice and palliative care. Thus, the first three years' data out of Oregon suggest that "hospice" and "hemlock" are not mutually exclusive, but may in some ways supplement or enhance one another. Whether the unique circumstances in Oregon can be duplicated in other states is an open, but eminently answerable, question.

Constance Putnam's book is important reading for those on both sides of the debate who are struggling with the potential compatibility of "hospice" and "hemlock." She presents a scholarly review of many of the underlying philosophical, ethical, and legal issues, and she combines this with summaries and anecdotes from personal interviews with several perceived leaders in both domains. The outstanding mix of sophisticated, well-researched thought and practical insight should make her book of interest both to scholars and to practitioners in the field of end-of-life care, as well as to laypersons who have struggled with these questions in their own lives. She ultimately decides that, in her view, compassion and self-determination are complementary and not incompatible. Her path to that conclusion is filled with ideas and information from which we all can benefit.

Timothy E. Quill, M.D.
Professor of Medicine, Psychiatry, and Medical Humanities
University of Rochester School of Medicine and Dentistry

Preface and Acknowledgments

Even before I began the research for this book, I knew I could not possibly do justice to all that has been written on how we die and how we think about it. There is, accordingly, much of relevance and importance that I have not discussed in my six chapters. But my aim in any case was never to cover the entire subject of death and dying. I have endeavored rather to pull together many strands from many fields, wanting above all to make a complicated, sensitive, and at times arcane subject accessible to a wide audience. This work is not meant to give answers, as such, but to serve as a guide to how one might go about finding one's own answers to some of the myriad questions that end-of-life decision-making provokes.

A few words about technical matters: All translations of words or phrases from foreign languages are mine. I have used the standard abbreviations of *NEJM* and *JAMA* for the *New England Journal of Medicine* and the *Journal of the American Medical Association* respectively; in the notes (though not in the text), I have abbreviated the *New York Times* and the *Boston Globe* as *NYT* and *BG,* and the *Hastings Center Report* as *HCR.* Other journal and newspaper names are for the most part written out; exceptions are the *BMJ* (as the *British Medical Journal* is now known) and, in the notes, some of the more easily recognizable or standardly abbreviated journals. Full citations are given the first time a work appears in each chapter; subsequent references are made with short titles only.

Thanks are due to many people. My thinking about Hospice and Hemlock, and about death and dying more generally, has been enormously enriched over the past decade by discussions with any and all who would open the door to me to talk about this difficult subject. Many were ready to do so, and I am grateful to them all. Without question the richest and most stimulating periods during all this work were the weeks I spent (more than once) at the Wellcome Institute for the History of Medicine in London (now the Wellcome Trust Centre for the History of Medicine at University College London), where the academic staff, resident and visiting scholars, and a dozen or more graduate students helped keep me on track and alert to the rich interdisciplinarity of my topic. Outside of London, Richard Andrews (then at Middlesex University) and Tony Walter (at the University of Reading) played especially important roles in helping me organize my thinking about the topic in the first place.

Over a period of several years, some half-dozen different colleagues have provided forums for me to present portions of my work; the ensuing discussions have always been helpful, and the content of the book has been improved as a result. Those who contributed to the book in this way are Vilhjálmur Árnason at the University of Reykjavík; Tony Walter at Reading University; Richard Andrews (now at York University) and Michael Bottery at Hull University; Jane Seymour at Sheffield University; Courtney Campbell at the University of Oregon; and Susan Stafford at Simmons College in Boston. Parts of the text are also based on papers I gave at two conferences of the International Society for the Study of Argumentation (ISSA) in Amsterdam and a presentation I made at a conference sponsored by the Netherlands Institute of Primary Health Care (NIVEL), also in Amsterdam. Discussants at each of these venues as well as colleagues who participated with me in a medical ethics delegation to China in 1995 further stimulated my thinking.

The five individuals I interviewed for the Profiles added much to my understanding of matters concerning Hospice and Hemlock, death and dying. In addition to the numerous persons to whose personal communications I refer in my notes, there is also a long list of family members, close friends, and acquaintances (exemplified by Kristin Ramsdell and Nancy Bedau, Sue Smyle and Luane Cole, and Dana Gelb Safran and—above all—Martine Cornelisse) who were willing not only to listen to me talk about death and dying but also to share their perspectives and their experiences, ideas, and reading matter. I am most particularly indebted to Dr. Louis B. Matthews, Jr., Dr. Sven M. Gundersen, and Harriet Adams Gundersen (all now deceased) who granted me the privilege of listening to their thoughts on dying as they sensed death approaching.

The following scholars from several different disciplines forced me to sharpen my thinking as each discussed one or more sections of the book with me, in several cases on more than one occasion: Margaret Battin, Hugo Bedau, Norman Daniels, Len Doyal, Martin Green, Clive Seale, Howard Solomon, and Judith Thomson. Miriam Graham Vasan believed in the book long before it saw its final form and worked with me to find a publisher.

My gratitude to all these people, named and unnamed, is great; equally great is my knowledge that I alone can be held responsible for the way I have used what I learned from each of them. If there are errors and if there is fuzzy thinking, the fault is mine. Having said that, I want also to make it a matter of record that the one who did the most to help me eliminate errors and fuzzy thinking is Hugo Bedau—husband, friend, and intellectual companion par excellence. He supported me from the outset and aided me in too many and too various ways for any mere acknowledgment of assistance to be adequate. Hence my dedication of the book to him.

Constance E. Putnam
Concord, Massachusetts
December 2001

1

The Matter of Death

Nothing should remain unsaid
At light snow's
Leading edge

—John Stearns Hayward[1]

From the dawn of life, death has been with us. Yet today, despite the fact that many still introduce their remarks about death and dying with a claim that it is a "taboo" subject,[2] we live in an age when discussions on these topics have become not only increasingly public but also more urgent. That urgency is a function of a wide range of social, medical, political, legal, and economic factors, among which the most prominent are the following: an aging population,[3] medical-technological innovations,[4] campaigns and referenda on physician-assisted suicide,[5] court decisions on physician-assisted suicide,[6] and rapidly rising health-care costs.[7]

Death matters to us for many reasons. If and when we begin thinking about dying, our thoughts are likely to take the form of wondering what it will be like for us personally to die. Who will be with us? What will our doctors (or other health-care providers) be able—or willing—to do on our behalf? My central concern in how we approach our dying is what we can expect from physicians, however, rather than from nurses (or other care-givers), precisely because the relationship with physicians is widely considered the more awkward of the two, the one more in need of revision and improvement. Several of the ways this relationship can suffer—or may need revision—are spelled out by physician Sidney H. Wanzer in his booklet *The End of Life: How to Deal with the System, A Practical Guide for Patients and Families* (2001). "These rights of [patients] and the obligations of physicians . . . are not always honored," he insists. Wanzer stresses the need for patients to know their rights and work with their physicians to make sure those rights are not violated.[8] This often-precarious relationship is the backdrop against which I intend the analysis of how we approach the crucial initial questions to be presented. In Chapter 5, I will face explicitly a few aspects of how to talk to one's doctor. By that time, I trust, some idea of what the questions are and how one ought to go about sorting them out will have been adequately answered.

I have aimed always to keep the patient's vantage point in the forefront. It is for this reason that I have sought to look at what constitutes "compassion" in a context when dying patients seek their physicians' help. Personal, anecdotal, literary, and professional evidence all indicate that high on the list of concerns is this: Dying people or those contemplating death (their own or another's) want above all for physicians to treat them with greater care than ever, to be present for them. (Fear of abandonment is a major source of concern, no doubt in part because tales of perceived abandonment are so commonplace.) They want to know that personal concern—compassion—rather than bureaucracy will guide health-care professionals' treatment of patients who have reached the end of the line.[9] This is precisely how physician Lonny Shavelson framed his moving portraits of five individuals confronting the possibility of assisted suicide. As he anticipated the death of his own parents, he made explicit the form he believes support from doctors and nurses needs to take: "I want at my side a hospice physician and nurse who will offer [my parents] the best of care. And if that is not enough, these health professionals should be able openly to arrange an injection that would provide my parents with the most merciful death."[10]

Although I have opted not to fill this work with personal anecdotes, part of my justification for the focus on compassion does, indeed, come not only from stories I have read (like Shavelson's) but also from personal experiences others have shared with me. I will mention three. A doctor's widow, years after her husband's death, still cannot quite believe the lack of compassion (her word) among her husband's professional colleagues—who abandoned him (again, her choice of words) as he lay dying. A twenty-something young woman and her family were treated brusquely and utterly without compassion—as she sees it—by the physicians caring for her father, who died when she was a teenager. A young man reports using his skills as a medic, skills he acquired in his military training, to "ease the passing" for his dying mother—because he believed it was the compassionate thing to do, and he could find no one else to help.

In short, "compassion" has seemed to me the word that best sums up the central point of what patients and their families want from their physicians.[11] An Episcopal minister in California put it this way: "When a terminally ill patient's suffering becomes intolerable despite every effort, this is a medical emergency that requires a compassionate response."[12] This is not at all to deny that many physicians already aim to offer just that to their patients. But what it means to be compassionate, what compassion is, turns out to be a difficult question to answer—surprisingly so, given the apparent general agreement that compassion is precisely what we want from our doctors.

I was initially prompted to think about this feature of the care we want from our doctors when we are dying by the felicitous phrase "heroic compassion," used by Sidney H. Wanzer and his colleagues in an important article that appeared in the *New England Journal of Medicine* (*NEJM*) in 1989. (The phrase occurs in a context that makes it clear the authors are playing it off against the tradition of "heroic measures," which calls up visions of dramatic last-minute medical or surgical interventions—not to mention television's *ER*.) Even when "aggressive curative techniques are no longer indicated," Wanzer and his colleagues wrote, "professionals and families are still called on to use intensive measures—extreme responsibility, extraordinary sensitivity, and heroic compassion."[13] This is the kind of intensive care most patients would love to have their doctors offer.

Based on this assumption that compassionate care is the goal, I will focus on what it is appropriate for the dying to expect, desire, or ask for by way of assistance from their physicians. The ground has been laid by those who say we must "contemplate what it means to live together as a compassionate society"[14] and that physicians and the public alike should "approach death together, not as adversaries, but as compassionate and enlightened friends."[15] Yet we must not forget that, for reasons patients often do not know or suspect, physicians may legitimately struggle with their own desire to be compassionate. Compassion does not always come easily.[16]

Along the way there are numerous intermediate questions to be asked, however, both about whether and why compassion is such a high priority and about what constitutes "heroic compassion." Some of the questions I raise I will respond to directly, but the purpose of this exercise is less to produce answers than to enable readers to figure out for themselves how to approach the questions and how to find their own answers. The issue, to re-iterate, is this: How does one begin thinking critically and systematically about the elusive, difficult, and anxiety-inducing questions that arise when we face death? What are the implications of what we *think* we think about these matters?

Two very different movements have grown up in recent decades, both directed at improving the lot of the dying and both laying claim—at least implicitly—to compassion. Indeed, a high percentage of the rhetoric about death and dying that bombards our society through the popular press is spawned by adherents of one or the other of these two movements, or by those who would attack the one or the other. The movements in question are what are often referred to as the "right-to-die movement" and the "hospice movement."

The "right-to-die movement" in the minds of many stands primarily for the right to commit suicide, though—as we will see—many related but different kinds of acts can be subsumed under the "right-to-die" heading. I have chosen to refer to this movement simply as "Hemlock" because of the way the poison hemlock (*Conium maculatum*) has been associated with death since classical times, as a prototype of a quick way out.[17] I shall also on occasion use the phrase "right to die"—essentially as a synonym—to describe this movement. A more common designation than "Hemlock" for the broader movement, actually quite widespread, "Right to Die" has begun to roll off the tongue with familiar ease. The expression is, however, fraught with difficulties of its own, as I will show.

The hospice movement, connected historically with places of respite for travelers in the Middle Ages (I will return to this topic in Chapter 2), I have chosen to refer to simply as "Hospice." Often touted as the ultimate expression of the move from "curing" to "caring," Hospice presents a view of how death should be approached that is in many respects diametrically opposed to that represented by Hemlock.[18]

Although the two movements are ostensibly concerned with the same issue (namely, how to assure that an individual's dying days are filled with as little misery and as much meaning as possible), they generally appear to be at loggerheads; their respective approaches to the dying process seem incompatible. Thoughtful people line up on both sides of the fence, with the result that those on the one side often are unable to see that those on the other side share their concern. Though strong rhetoric at times makes the fence appear to be an impenetrable barrier, it is my hope that better understanding will show a way through the fence. Much is to be gained in the alleviation of human suffering if the wisdom on both sides can be put to work; learning how to think more clearly about the matters at hand seems eminently worth the effort.

The one absolutely inevitable fact of our lives, once we have been born, is our deaths—which is the experience we are least able to understand fully. If a doctor who said he was reflecting "on a life of dealing with death and dying" was right in being persuaded "that death's anguish is, in no small measure, man made . . . a product of Western culture," then it is perhaps this peculiarly Western inability to grasp death or give "death its due," that makes it appear ominous.[19] Whether this in turn makes death necessarily an evil has long been a matter of debate. Historian Philippe Ariès, for example, has amassed considerable evidence that death has by no means always been feared or always been seen as evil. In the Middle Ages, he tells us, there was a development "of a sensibility that assigned . . . high value" to physical death; it was not until later that "[m]oralists, the religious, and mendicant friars exploited the new anxiety." Death might "not yet have been causing fear, [but] it was causing uncertainty."[20] And while that is not equivalent to death being seen as evil, a move in the direction of that view had begun to take place. Even so, we should not forget that there are religious and cultural traditions today in which death is more celebrated than feared, in which "death is the opening, the portal, not the end."[21]

Historically, a strong thread woven into debates about death has been that we have nothing to fear about death because we no longer exist once death claims us. Epicurus, in ancient Greece, is perhaps still the most persuasive spokesperson for this idea: "So death, the most terrifying of ills, is nothing to us, since so long as we exist death is not with us; but when death comes, then we do not exist."[22] Some two centuries later, in Rome, Lucretius echoed that sentiment: "From all of this it follows that *death is nothing to us* and no concern of ours. . . . So, when we shall be no more— when the union of body and spirit that engenders us has been disrupted— to us, who shall then be nothing, nothing by any hazard will happen any more at all."[23]

Others, however, have argued seriously and cogently that death is indeed evil. Philosopher Fred Feldman takes pains to analyze the Epicurean view that death is of no import and therefore cannot be evil, and he concludes that it *is* evil, though not *self-evidently* so. Most importantly, it is evil for the one who is dead.[24] Daniel Callahan, another philosopher, discusses death as an evil both more subtly and more persuasively in *The Troubled Dream of Life: Living with Mortality* (1993). Of particular importance to him is the distinction he draws between death as a biological evil and death as a moral evil.[25]

More common are various insistences that death is, if not exactly evil, nonetheless something to be feared. Writer and philosopher Simone de Beauvoir tells us that what makes us fear death is that it "puts an end to [one's] drive." Cut off from his "transcendence . . . an individual is nothing; it is by his projects that he fulfills himself."[26] Perceived this way, death of course makes us fearful; it is a complete nullification of our projects. Ernest Becker (trained originally as an anthropologist) went further. Preferring to speak of the "terror" of death, he insists in his book *The Denial of Death* (1973) that when this terror seems to have disappeared, it is rather the case that it has been (however temporarily) repressed, or denied.[27] By cutting off the possibility of any future, death threatens constantly to deprive us of life's meaning. Physician Joanne Lynn would have us believe that "[d]ying serves to make life more precious and personal issues more pressing."[28] Clearly, death matters to us.

So there death sits—or, less benignly, there it looms—out in front of us somewhere, waiting and watching for us. Where daily experience gives us the illusion of understanding life at least some of the time, death is wholly elusive. Furthermore, we learn little about our own death from anyone else's. Death is the most solitary of experiences. Yet, facing (or denying or preparing for) this lonely event of dying is inextricably woven into the fabric of our lives. How we live affects how we die, and how we think about dying affects the way we live.[29] Worse yet, dying today appears to be particularly complex, leaving many people confused and anxious.

Despite the difficulties, however, there has been enormous growth recently in thanatology (death studies).[30] Moreover, there is a burgeoning literature on death and dying, one of several indications that death is less a taboo subject than it was in the not-so-distant past. In 1994, an article on the way death has "wormed its way into the world of marketing, inspiring a number of macabre products," had a subhead under its title "Death Wishes" pronouncing boldly: "All of a sudden, the subject of dying is no longer taboo."[31] More recently, another writer referred to the plethora of books on death in a lighthearted manner. "Let's all share a sardonic chuckle over this cosmic paradox," he wrote. "At the height of its global ascendancy, supposedly optimistic and youth-obsessed America is now also increasingly fixated on death."[32]

Even so, the subject of death is surely still taboo in the sense that it is not only an uncomfortable one for most individuals, but also one that is considered inappropriate for casual conversations in most ordinary social settings. Few people are really eager to take up the imponderables of this unavoidable aspect of the human condition.[33] Among those who, in recent decades, have helped focus attention on the relevance and value of discussing death are several writers whose books have clarified for a wide range of readers both why it is that death matters so much and what some of the features are that bother us about death and dying. Certainly a point could be made for giving breakthrough status to Herman Feifel's *The Meaning of Death,* which was published in 1959 and generated sufficient interest for *Time* magazine to review it.[34] The result, it has been said, was that for "the first time in decades, Americans could pick up a popular periodical and read a levelheaded discussion of dying and death on the contemporary scene."[35]

In 1974, Ernest Becker won the Pulitzer Prize for general non-fiction for his *Denial of Death,* a probing analysis of how fear of death dominates life. The book is filled with references to and quotations from a stunning array of scholars, but Becker does a remarkable job of making a difficult subject accessible. Even those who knew little about psychoanalysis, or merely read about the book (or heard it being discussed), probably benefited from being exposed perhaps for the first time to the centrality in human life of the very human fear of death.

Similarly, nearly a decade earlier—and thus only a few years after Feifel's book—sociologists Barney G. Glaser and Anselm L. Strauss had explored the context in which hospital patients were doing their dying.

Their book, *Awareness of Dying* (1965), was an intensely academic project, however; a central concern for them was that Americans, while willing and able to talk about specific deaths (witness the newspaper headlines, they tell us[36]), were generally unwilling to think in the abstract about death or the dying process. The result, they contended, was that doctors and other health-care providers also had difficulty developing adequate strategies for coping with their dying patients.

The book that had the most dramatic and, as it has turned out, lasting effect on the way a great many people think about what happens once an individual develops an "awareness of dying" was Elisabeth Kübler-Ross's *On Death and Dying* (1969). Never out of print in the more than thirty years since it was initially published, this book is more frequently mentioned than any other as the one that opened discussion of death and dying to the general populace, the one that started a revolution.[37]

At least two factors made *On Death and Dying* both different and important. First, Kübler-Ross looked at dying from the patient's point of view; her concern was how dying persons themselves react to the news of their diagnosis and then to the experience of dying. Second, Kübler-Ross anticipated Ernest Becker by identifying the inclination among the dying to deny their imminent death. But where Becker concentrated on the denial that stems from fear of dying, Kübler-Ross discovered (and reported) that dying patients typically go through several emotional stages; denial is only one of them. Her straightforward analysis of the five (now famous) "stages" through which she found those who are dying typically go gave Kübler-Ross's work its prominence. Many who have never read (or perhaps even heard of) her book will nonetheless talk about "stages" in this context—often with quotation marks (literal or figurative), as if they are vaguely aware of relying on someone else's idea. "The five stages of dying" has become part of the argot, though denial, anger, depression, bargaining, and acceptance are of course not stages of dying as such. Instead, they mark the changes in emotions that dying individuals are apt to undergo. The insight that patients may go through phases was perceptive; unfortunately, many people have interpreted the five stages as a rigidly descriptive sequence. In reality, the experience of dying is rarely so neat, and by no means do all dying persons pass through all five stages.[38]

Another book that apparently resonated with a great many readers was Jessica Mitford's *The American Way of Death* (1963). Actually less about death and dying than it was about the expensive way in which Americans are wont to deal with funerals and burials, the book detailed these matters in a way that showed how some of the costs are a direct outcome of a peculiarly American fear of dying. The unwillingness to talk about death results, Mitford insisted, in a special form of death denial.[39] Among the contributions Mitford made in this book—quite apart from the enmity she aroused among funeral directors for what amounted to an exposé of the funeral industry—was that she helped people think and talk about death more openly than had previously been common. Unquestionably, Mitford's book stimulated discussion of the *business* of dying, opening the 1960s to a new attitude toward the subject.

Others, subsequently, have written books on one aspect or another of death, some of which have had a surprising degree of popularity. How much credit for this increase in interest is owed to the authors just cited— Becker, Glaser and Strauss, Kübler-Ross, Mitford—is difficult to say. Certainly in the 1990s, three additional very different books in the death-and-dying genre that garnered widespread attention when they appeared give strong evidence that the topic is with us to stay. In 1993, Daniel Callahan published his extraordinarily thoughtful *Troubled Dream of Life* (mentioned earlier). A year later, in Holland, Bert Keizer published a book called *Het refrein is Hein* (which translates as "Rounds with the Grim Reaper"). The wild popularity of this young physician-author's reflections on death spurred him to translate it into English; it appeared first in England and then (in 1997) in the United States under an altered title, *Dancing with Mister D: Notes on Life and Death*.[40] Shortly before that, the Yale surgeon Sherwin B. Nuland put his populist pen to work on *How We Die: Reflections on Life's Final Chapter* (1994), a book that enjoyed dramatic commercial success from the outset (and won the National Book Award).[41] Nuland claimed too much credit for his own role in the "death awareness" movement when he mused in an interview that "what I seem to have done is start a movement of national consciousness."[42] Still, the length of time his book stayed on the best-seller list is one of the strongest hints to date that many people are willing to think in more specific detail about death— their own and that of others.

These volumes constitute but a small fraction of the books concerned with death and dying that are available to readers today. The large number of volumes on the subject, some of them very successful and others less widely read but with a devoted following, is a clear sign of contemporary interest in and concern about the general subject. Nor are books with close ties to the dominant culture the only ones being read. For years, *The Tibetan Book of the Dead* has had quasi-cult status, particularly among young people and those with an eye on alternative lifestyles and holistic approaches to life and death.[43] Less trendy, but a book that also speaks to a sometimes disaffected audience looking for help outside the mainstream, is *Dying, Death, and Bereavement: Theoretical Perspectives and Other Ways of Knowing* (1994).[44] That book's chief value lies in the way it engages in cross-cultural exploration of the experience of death.

If death and dying had not changed so significantly in recent years as a result (among other things) of the factors mentioned above—the graying of the population, skyrocketing health-care costs, and (especially) medical-technological progress—the persistent resistance to facing death squarely might not matter so much. But the truth is that dying has become harder, not easier, in contemporary society. Decisions are now called for where once there were no options and thus nothing to decide. The one positive thing to be said about the inevitability of death, in the past, was that decisions and actions were largely taken out of one's hands. There was nothing one could do about death (in most cases); it came or it did not—and sooner or later, of course, it did. Today, at least the illusion exists that there is a lot one can do. What was previously perhaps unpleasant or undesirable (it may well still be that) is now something that must also be pondered, thought about, dealt with, confronted, decided on.

The literature helps. But much of what has been written leaves important questions unanswered. The personal stories that serve as the leitmotiv or fill the pages of many books are rich resources; they bring us close to real persons who have had real experiences with death and dying.[45] To be sure, telling stories is a time-honored way of getting ideas across and explaining complex issues, and anecdotes about someone else's dying will almost certainly tear at our heartstrings, inspire us, or alert us to experiences we hope to avoid. But the agony your grandmother endured because her doctor would not prescribe enough pain medication, the wonderful care your neighbor received from a particular Hospice nurse, the family fight that ensued when you and your siblings tried to decide what was best for your dying father, the heartbreaking tale of a premature baby whose life was just beyond sustaining—none of these stories tells me how to begin thinking about my own death. And in the end, what concerns each of us most is the first-person-singular story: *my* dying, *my* death.

Philosophical debates in the professional literature on the definition of death, the rights of patients to refuse unwanted treatments, or how "quality of life" is to be measured are useful exercises when the aim is to expand knowledge and understanding. For the most part, however, despite their merits, these discussions remain remote and do not reach the general public. Much the same can be said about the medical and ethical questions raised in journals read by physicians: What do professional standards require of physicians whose patients are dying? What does it mean to act in a manner consistent with the "integrity of the profession"? What role does (or should) the inherent uncertainty of medical knowledge play in a doctor's thinking?[46] What counts as "futile" treatment? How much of this can (or should) be conveyed to patients? Is the doctor who assists in a patient's dying guilty of helping to "kill" that patient? What is written by and for doctors on such issues remains accessible largely only to doctors themselves. The rest of us know little about what doctors really think.

The exact status of the law on suicide (physician assisted or otherwise) and additional legal issues around the dying of patients tend to be taken up primarily in legal and medical journals. Only fragmentary discussions on these matters appear in the daily papers. Detailed analyses of whether physician-assisted suicide ought to be legalized and careful explication of the laws relating to how physicians should treat their dying patients (and who should make the decisions) appear primarily in publications not read by the average dying citizen and not understood much beyond the confines of the legal fraternity.

Of course, newspaper reporters and columnists do cover these issues. Dr. Jack Kevorkian, with his "suicide machine" and macabre self-promotion has been a veritable fount of news copy. Whether Holland is really a medically sanctioned killing ground and whether the voters of Oregon have paved a smooth road to legalized killing by doctors seem to be perennial favorites of op-ed writers. The time and space constraints under which newspaper writers work, however, mean that the analyses of these important medical, ethical, and legal questions are almost always superficial. Newspaper columns simply do not permit discussions of the length and depth that the issues merit. Thus the information most readily accessible to the proverbial man or woman in the street—or hospital, nursing home, or Hospice bed—is at best incomplete.

Furthermore, most people do not read the newspaper in the reflective and thoughtful mood that the subject of death (especially one's own) warrants. What makes good copy or dramatic headlines may very well not indicate the state of the art in current thinking on what is arguably one of the most important subjects in contemporary society. Ordinary men and women do push beyond the obvious to find more thorough discussions, as the startling success of some of the death-and-dying titles mentioned above indicates, but clearly no one has time or energy to read them all. In any case, most books and articles turn out to be either too general or too specific (too impersonal or, ironically, too personal), too narrowly professional and difficult to understand, too short to plumb the depths adequately or too long and detailed to absorb and retain. Little or nothing of what has been written at book length helps the curious and concerned individual with the crucial initial questions: Where should I begin thinking about my death? How should I approach the topic? What issues are relevant and important for me to make decisions about? The desire to help fill that gaping hole is the motivating force behind all of what fills the following pages.[47]

Many of the topics that have appeared in professional journals (and that are certainly relevant to "death studies") will be conspicuous by their relative absence from my discussion, however. Some I will mention in passing, a way of acknowledging that they are part of the larger issue; some I will discuss more briefly than their significance for many persons warrants. The rationale behind such apparent omissions is straightforward: First things should come first. I am convinced that for most people the primary issue (in the literal sense) is not a philosophically impeccable definition of death, for instance. Neither is it what religion teaches about suicide or what the legal status of physician-assisted suicide is in every jurisdiction. And it certainly is not the point at which physicians may legally and ethically—and with medical efficacy—remove organs from dying patients for purposes of transplant. It is, rather, "What is my dying apt to be like and what can or should I do about it?"

What I have said so far is not intended to be a full-scale explanation of *why* the topic of death matters, but it should suffice to validate the claim that death and dying *do* matter to human beings. Philosopher Ronald Dworkin, in a book to which I shall return, puts it eloquently: Death not only matters, it has *dominion*. And death "has dominion," he says, "because it is not only the start of nothing but the end of everything."[48]

That scholarly and very appropriate observation notwithstanding, the headline-grabbers in recent years, on matters having to do with death and dying in the United States, fall into two categories of a rather different sort. The first comprises Dr. Jack Kevorkian's activities on behalf of the dying (as he would have it) and his travails with the law. The second—although it is related, there are important reasons for keeping it distinct—is the series of political and legal battles, accompanied by considerable discussion, over the appropriateness of legalizing physician-assisted suicide. Newspaper and magazine articles, book chapters and whole books could be (and have been) written on one or both of these topics, or on subtopics within one or both of them.

With all of this, a major question that had been slowly emerging from behind the ivy-covered walls of academe has abruptly appeared on center stage in very public theaters. Do we have a "right to die," a right to do whatever it takes to alleviate unremitting pain and with it therefore to use "hemlock" (metaphorically speaking) or at least to have access to it? Virtually in lockstep with the growing interest in this matter—in part influenced by discussions around the subject and in part by fear that the answer might be affirmative—another issue has arisen. The rather abstract and philosophical questions of whether we human beings should be allowed to exercise control over how much we have to suffer and of when and how we die (which includes whether physician-assisted suicide should be legalized) cannot stand alone. Both Kevorkian's methods of assisting patients to die and less controversial (or medically more mainstream) methods have helped sharpen interest in whether there are ways dying patients can be helped other than by hastening their deaths.

Enter Hospice. As more and more dying persons and their families have benefited from the supportive, family-centered, team-of-caregivers approach to alleviating the pain and suffering that often accompany dying, Hospice as an alternative has gained considerable media attention.[49] Indeed, "hospice care" has become a regular part of the vocabulary of all those who care for the dying or are engaged in "death studies"—even when it is not a Hospice organization strictly speaking that is involved.[50] Meanwhile, saying someone is in "hospice care" has become a coded means of indicating that the person in question is dying.

Yet in a nation where nearly two and a half million persons die annually, fewer than half a million persons are typically receiving Hospice care in a given year. In other words, by no means do all of those who are dying avail themselves of Hospice care—either because they are not interested, there is no Hospice close at hand, or they do not "qualify." Hospice has filled an important niche for at least some of the "actively dying," but it is "limited to patients who have been diagnosed as having a 'terminal illness' with six months or fewer to live and is generally focused on cancer and AIDS patients."[51] Thus Hospice can hardly be the whole answer, though it does offer a clear alternative to having doctors directly help their patients die. One of the underlying premises of greatest import in official Hospice circles is that nothing should be done that will intentionally either delay *or* hasten the natural dying process.[52] Thus suicide is a non-option for those dying under Hospice care, and physician-assisted suicide and euthanasia are explicitly ruled out.

Why look at Hospice (in the broadest sense of that term) on the one hand and the possibility of Hemlock (the right to die that may include the idea of physician assistance in dying) on the other, rather than at some more middle-of-the-road medical approaches to the dying? Hospice, with its strong emphasis on palliation—the national organization's change of name from "National Hospice Organization" to "National Hospice and Palliative Care Organization" in February 2000 is a strong indicator of this—has been in the forefront of contemporary efforts to improve care for the dying and is thus an obvious choice.[53] Hemlock—the term I will use to refer generically to the multitude of efforts (including Kevorkian's) loosely subsumed under the "right to die" rubric—with its cries for choice, control, and self-determination—at least appears to raise a direct challenge to Hospice. Some, maybe most, of the adherents of Hospice and of Hemlock stand at opposite ends of the continuum with respect to how it is appropriate for human beings to act as they approach the end of life. Even so, there is considerable territory between the extremes defined by Hospice and Hemlock, and numerous positions could be plotted along that continuum.[54]

One thing we need to get straight first is what language we will use to describe the activity central to my discussion, namely, the act or acts engaged in by a physician to help a patient die. I prefer to speak of "physician aid in dying" rather than "physician-assisted suicide" (PAS). Not least of the reasons is that this makes possible an explicit parallel to "physician aid in living," something we can surely all agree we want from our doctors. To speak of "physician assistance in dying" or of "assisted dying" (an expression Dr. Timothy Quill likes to use—see my Profile of him in Chapter 4) can help open the discussion for those tempted to turn their backs on any discussion of "euthanasia" and "physician-assisted suicide."

Another possibility of a similar sort would be to talk of "physician support in dying." The emphasis in this phrase might more easily be seen as referring to positive behavior on the part of the physician, over a period of time, rather than as something as simple and direct as aid at the end of that process.[55] To the extent that "physician support in dying" helps us focus on the dying *process* rather than the death *event,* it might well be an improvement. Seeing "physician aid" and "physician support" as rough equivalents, however, I shall use both. For clarity's sake, I will avoid acronyms altogether, including the widely used "PAS."

Finally, a few words about four of the topics—very different in nature—that I will not be dealing with at length, despite their importance in popular thinking about death and dying and in my own views on the subject. I wish to clarify why I am not giving them more substantial treatment. These are: definitions of death, the role of religion, the concept of medical futility, and the very difficult and troubling problems that arise when the dying patient is incompetent.

Take the last of these first. "Incompetence" can be used to refer to those who are incompetent either congenitally or by reason of age, or rendered so by the progression of the disease; thus an individual of once-considerable mental competence who has lost the capacity for rationality is also covered by the term. Needless to say, such individuals are by definition not able to make rational decisions for themselves, and hence they must rely on the good will of others to make decisions for them. A second (often related) group of persons thought to be especially vulnerable are the elderly.[56] Not to discuss such cases is a significant omission; certainly there are writers who argue that unless or until we can cope with the difficult cases, we have made little progress in deciding how end-of-life decisions are to be made. The position I take rests on an argument running in the other direction: If we cannot even deal with the "easy" cases, what hope is there for being able to manage the "difficult" ones? Three clinicians who have wrestled with all these matters devised a set of clinical criteria for physician-assisted suicide for "hopelessly ill" patients. But despite acknowledging that "patients should not be held hostage to our reluctance or inability to forge policies," they admit that their proposed criteria exclude patients who fit the bill (including having mental competence) *except for being physically able to act on their own.*[57] In other words, these well-established experts in the field have taken a "let's deal with the easy cases first" approach. I am disinclined to second-guess them while we are in what must still be considered early days in the debate over the legalization of physician-assisted suicide or other forms of physician-aid-in-dying.

Let us turn now to the other three topics I said I would exclude from any full-scale discussion. The first of these is how to define death. Superficially, it might seem that we all know what death is. As Fred Feldman has pointed out, "According to a popular view, there is nothing mysterious about death—it is just the cessation of life."[58] But he then goes on to acknowledge that "death is problematic in very many different ways." He proceeds to list as examples eight categories of "questions about death" that need exploration if one is truly to understand death or be able to explain what it is. Psychological, legal, biological, theological, literary, sociological, economic, and medical features all appear on the landscape of potential analysis as Feldman paints it.[59]

Philippe Ariès, in the masterful work of his mentioned earlier on the way Western attitudes toward death have changed through the millennium, drew attention to another way of defining death when he coined the expression "tame death."[60] Ariès was in many ways more concerned with *dying* than with *death,* as Daniel Callahan explains when he says that the contrast to "tame death" is a "wild death [that] is not only a technological death, but a hidden, dirty death, one that is shunned, feared, and denied." It is the *dying process* as much as the death itself to which the adjectives apply.[61]

Despite the way a definition of death obviously is connected with my topic of what it is appropriate for dying patients to expect (or ask for) in the way of assistance from their physicians, I intend for the most part to ignore the issue. There are at least two reasons for putting this controversial topic to one side. The first is that I am far more concerned with the *approach* it is appropriate for people to make toward death (when they are not caught unprepared or unawares by death) than I am with death itself. I see "dying" as a *process* and "death" as an *event*. Facing that dying process—what transpires on the path that leads to death, and how we can or do or should behave in the midst of the journey along that path—is my subject. The end, death itself, I take as a given and not as something to be analyzed or discussed.

The second reason for ignoring definitions of death is that, simply put, people by and large do not worry about defining death. For most ordinary people under ordinary circumstances, dead is dead, the result of a natural process. Those who are dying and their families alike generally know both that death is imminent and when it has come. In many cases they catch the signals before the physicians and other caretakers are prepared to make any pronouncement.[62] Sometimes dying persons gather their families around them when they sense "the end is near" (as my mother did). Alternatively, the dying stop eating or shrink within themselves, becoming more withdrawn and seeming to fade away (which happened with my mother-in-law). Others utterly lose the capacity for communication, so that all concerned know the person is in a very real sense no longer there (here, too, I have an example from my own life—the dying of my friend, Bud Harmon). Or (to take an example from literature), like Milly Theale in Henry James's *Wings of the Dove,* they simply turn their faces to the wall.[63] That turning may be literal, as in Milly's case, or it may be metaphorical. Nothing important depends on which it is.

If I am right that most people "know" when death has come, or know how to tell that it is imminent, then—for a discussion of how to negotiate one's way through the dying process—we do not need to debate conflicting definitions of death. This is not to deny the value of continuing the discussion elsewhere.[64] But if the issue hasn't been settled yet, despite the many experts who have spilled so much ink on it, a few paragraphs or even a chapter here will not do the trick. I do not want this difficult subject to distract us from my main concern, which is this: How do we best traverse the terrain that lies between where we are now and where we will be when death comes, and what approach is likely to surround us most satisfactorily with compassion?

Finally, religion is another topic I have set largely to one side. This is not so easy, given the extent to which issues related to death and dying seem for many to be inextricably intertwined with religious beliefs and sentiments. Indeed, for many religions it could perhaps fairly be said that the central issues are precisely what death means and how death is to be faced. Religion can itself be seen as first and foremost an attempt to explain the human condition in the face of human mortality.

But among the reasons for trying to put religion and religious views about death and dying to one side is the way careful, rational discussion can be undercut when any discussant invokes God. Religious teachings, however important they may be for numerous individuals, cannot be central to general social policy in a liberal democratic society. Steering away from faith-based discussions about death and dying is thus critical. We live in a diverse and largely sectarian society; what follows from sectarian beliefs in one tradition may very well be irrelevant in another. Second, religious beliefs are (as I implied above) often—strictly speaking—irrational; that is, they are based on tradition or faith or the authority of a religious hierarchy rather than on logical analysis and scientific endeavor. Religious views on how it is appropriate for dying persons to behave as they approach their own death frequently rely on an appeal to the deity that limits further discussion. Once God is invoked, there is nothing more to say.[65]

Having said all this, however, I would not dispute that attitudes toward death may be affected by religious sentiments or that attempts to give room to the spiritual dimensions of life may prove beneficial to some dying persons. To the extent that this is so for particular individuals, they will surely want to include considerations of religious or spiritual matters in whatever self-assessments they make of the trajectory of their lives (a point to which I will return in Chapter 5).

A final subject of considerable importance and direct relevance that I will touch on only briefly is the way end-of-life decisions frequently center around a determination of whether the care that might be extended to the patient is "futile." Immediately questions arise as to what "futility" really means and whether the only kind of futility that needs consideration is "medical" futility. Doctors and patients might well disagree. As was pointed out in a study of just such conflicts between physicians' practices and patients' wishes, however, even though "futility is not a new concept in medicine, defining its practical implications represents a new social and clinical frontier."[66]

Central to the difficulty in talking about "futility" in a medical context, as more than one writer has stressed, is that it sounds so clear and final that people are easily misled into thinking they know exactly what it means. The "word 'futile' has a categorical ring that masks a more subtle complexity," writes American doctor Stuart J. Youngner.[67] He is echoed by British physician John Saunders: "Futility has an air of finality, a ring of clarity, an echo of facts fighting back against values. . . . The notion of futility is certainly not the simple one it is intended to imply."[68] Others tell us "[s]imple statements of futility are inherently incomplete, being ambiguous with respect to the goals of treatment and vague with respect to the probability of success."[69]

On the other hand, at least some members of the medical profession think they do understand "futility" well enough to know that it is what allows them to make decisions (apparently unilaterally) about whether, for example, to administer cardiopulmonary resuscitation (CPR) for a patient at the end of life who has gone into cardiac arrest: "[M]ost doctors and nurses believe that there are some patients for whom resuscitation in the event of cardiopulmonary arrest would be inappropriate for reasons of futility or poor quality of life. Clinical teams can exclude these patients from resuscitation attempts," we are told in a report of a British survey of do-not-resuscitate orders.[70] Three American writers on the subject are more blunt: "[F]utility is a professional judgment that takes precedence over patient autonomy."[71]

What compounds the difficulty in coming to grips with the concept of futility is that it turns out there are numerous kinds of futility; "medical futility" is only one way to express part of what can be meant by the term. Nancy S. Jecker, for instance, urging that "we should think about the term 'futility' as marking a point along a probability continuum," reminds us that it is helpful to distinguish between quantitative futility and qualitative futility.[72] John Saunders, whom I quoted above, additionally lists "cognitive" and "physiological" futility (the latter he calls "absolute").[73] A thorough analysis of these variant ways of looking at futility is beyond the scope of this project, but it should at least be clear that futility is not a unitary concept. If there is more than one kind of futility, it stands to reason that there is more than one kind of answer to questions having to do with when or whether it is appropriate to designate a particular form of therapy as futile.

With these qualifications and exclusions behind us, I turn at last to pose more precisely the thematic question of this book: To what extent do Hospice and Hemlock, separately or together, adequately reflect values held to be central in contemporary U.S. society—and do these movements (again, separately or together) give adequate room for physicians to exercise the compassion toward their dying patients that those patients seem concerned to receive? An alternative way of putting the question somewhat more personally might be this: How does one figure out what it is appropriate for dying patients to expect by way of help from their physicians, and can either Hospice or Hemlock alone provide that?

NOTES

1. John Stearns Hayward, from "When the wind blows . . ." in *Energy* (Ithaca, N.Y.: [privately published], 1997), [n.p.].

2. See, e.g., "[D]eath is a taboo subject in our culture . . . we both deny and fear it." Derek Humphry and Mary Clement, *Freedom to Die: People, Politics, and the Right-to-Die Movement* (New York: St. Martin's Press, 1998), p. 21. Earlier, Linda Emanuel (of the American Medical Association's Institute for Ethics) was quoted in a call-out at the head of a newspaper article saying, "Death is a taboo. The medical profession is very tender about the subject because our whole society is very tender about it." Richard A. Knox, "End-of-life care fuels a nascent discussion," *BG* (27 June 1997): A17.

3. The U.S. Bureau of the Census, *Statistical Abstract of the United States: 1998* (a.k.a. "The National Data Book"), 118th ed. (Washington, D.C., 1998): 15 (Table No. 14) shows the over-85 population growing from less than 1 percent of the total U.S. population in 1980 to 1.5 percent of the total population in the year 2000.

4. Examples include respirators, dialysis machines, organ transplants, and various other procedures (such as intubating comatose patients to deliver nutrition and hydration), which enable a particular human life to be supported beyond its natural limit.

5. Washington and California both narrowly defeated bills that would have legalized physician-assisted suicide (in 1991 and 1992, respectively) before Oregon passed such a bill in 1994. More recently, lawmakers in Maine and Michigan rejected similar laws (in February and November 1998, respectively). See "Maine Lawmakers Reject Bill Allowing Doctors Assisted Suicides," *NYT* (12 Feb. 1998): A25.

6. Most significant are the Supreme Court rulings in *Washington v. Glucksberg* and *Vacco v. Quill*. See the series of articles in *NYT* (27 June 1997): A1, A18–A19; see also Ronald Dworkin, Thomas Nagel, Robert Nozick, et al., "Assisted Suicide: The Philosophers' Brief" (an amicus brief filed in these Supreme Court cases), *The New York Review* (27 Mar. 1997): 41–47, and Dworkin's "Assisted Suicide: What the Court Really Said," *The New York Review* (25 Sept. 1997): 40, 42–43, written after the decision was handed down.

7. Physician Joanne Lynn (see my Profile of her in Ch. 5), as vigorous an advocate for better care of the dying as there is, has remarked that our health-care system is one "where people are routinely bankrupted by the costs of long-term care." See "Should Doctors Hasten Death?" *Dartmouth Med.* 17, no. 1 (Fall 1992): 39. Another cost of dying—that of the cost of funerals—is also a subject of widespread concern. Costs in the Boston area in 2001 could range from less than $1,000 for "direct cremation" to well more than $6,000 for a traditional funeral with full service from the funeral director. I am indebted to Ted Tunnicliffe of MacRae-Tunnicliffe Funeral Home in Concord, Massachusetts, for these rough figures.

8. Sidney H. Wanzer, *The End of Life: How to Deal with the System, A Practical Guide for Patients and Families* (Denver, Colo.: The Hemlock Society, 2001), pp. 6, 17.

9. In spelling out what they call "The Argument from Compassion," Martin Gunderson and David J. Mayo, "Restricting Physician-Assisted Death to the Terminally Ill," *HCR* 30, no. 6 (Nov.-Dec. 2000): 18, say that "Compassion is often cited as a reason for physician-assisted death."

10. Lonny Shavelson, *A Chosen Death: The Dying Confront Assisted Suicide* (New York: Simon & Schuster, 1995), p. 232. He did not get his wish, as the tale of his father's death in the "Afterword" of the updated paperback edition shows (Berkeley: University of California Press, 1998), pp. 232–35.

11. A fine example of the importance of "compassion" to doctors and patients alike appears in an article about Dr. Matthew Warpick, a quintessential family doctor who was still practicing in New York City at the age of 90. Warpick is quoted saying, "There's a word in Yiddish called *rachmones.* . . . Loosely translated, it means compassion. I've tried to treat all my patients with compassion, and, as a result, they've become good friends." Michael Ryan, "Doctor, Don't Retire," *Parade Mag.* (27 Oct. 1997): 18.

12. Cecil McIver, *Assisted Dying as a Moral and Ethical Choice: A Physician's View* (Denver, Colo.: The Hemlock Society, 2000), p. 15.

13. Sidney H. Wanzer, Daniel D. Federman, S. James Adelstein, et al., "The Physician's Responsibility Toward Hopelessly Ill Patients: A Second Look," *NEJM* 320, no. 13 (30 Mar. 1989): 47.

14. Barbara Supanich and Howard Brody, "Ethical Issues Concerning Physician-Assisted Death," insist that there is agreement about care in 97 percent of the cases but that open dialogue is needed for the rest, in John F. Monagle and David C. Thomasma, eds., *Health Care Ethics: Critical Issues for the 21st Century* (Gaithersburg, Md.: Aspen Publishers, 1998), p. 309.

15. Sandol Stoddard, *The Hospice Movement: A Better Way of Caring for the Dying* (New York: Vintage, 1992 [1978]), p. 7. See also Robert Wirthnow, *Acts of Compassion: Caring for Others and Helping Ourselves* (Princeton, N.J.: Princeton University Press, 1991).

16. "Compassion is not something we can turn off and on," wrote a Jewish doctor as she laid out the challenge she faced when she found herself caring for an unreconstructed Nazi patient. "Do we develop compassion only if the patient is morally, philosophically acceptable to us?" Renate G. Justin, "Can a Physician Always Be Compassionate?" *HCR* 30, no. 4 (July-Aug. 2000): 27.

17. The death of Socrates sets the stage for all other references to hemlock as a means of death. The standard account of what drinking the hemlock was actu-

ally like—Socrates's last minutes and his taking of the poison ("quite calmly and with no sign of distaste, he drained the cup in one breath")—appears in Plato's "Phaedo," in Edith Hamilton and Huntington Cairns, eds., *Plato: The Collected Dialogues* (New York: Pantheon Books, 1961), p. 97.

18. On the contrast between Hospice and Hemlock for critically ill patients, see, e.g., J. Curtis and G. Rubenfield, eds., *Managing Death in the ICU: The Transition from Cure to Comfort* (New York: Oxford University Press, 2000).

19. Bernard Lown, *The Lost Art of Healing* (Boston: Houghton Mifflin, 1996), p. 288.

20. Philippe Ariès (Helen Weaver, trans.), *The Hour of Our Death* (New York: Oxford University Press, 1991 [Knopf, 1981]), pp. 297, 298.

21. Lee Palmer Wandel, introduction to "Framing Death: Cultural and Religious Responses," in Howard M. Spiro, Mary G. McCrea Curnen, and Lee Palmer Wandel, eds., *Facing Death: Where Culture, Religion, and Medicine Meet* (New Haven, Conn.: Yale University Press, 1996), p. 111.

22. Epicurus, "Letter to Menoeceus," in Whitney J. Oates, ed. (C. Bailey, trans.), *The Stoic and Epicurean Philosophers* (New York: Modern Library, 1957 [1940]), p. 31.

23. Lucretius (R. E. Latham, trans.), *The Nature of the Universe* (Harmondsworth, England: Penguin, 1951), p. 121.

24. Fred Feldman, *Confrontations with the Reaper: A Philosophical Study of the Nature and Value of Death* (New York: Oxford University Press, 1992), pp. 127–56.

25. Daniel Callahan, *The Troubled Dream of Life: Living with Mortality* (New York: Simon & Schuster, 1993), pp. 174–86 and generally.

26. Simone de Beauvoir (Bernard Frechtman, trans.), *The Ethics of Ambiguity* (New York: Philosophical Library, 1948), pp. 107, 115.

27. Ernest Becker, *The Denial of Death* (New York: Free Press, 1973), p. 15 and generally.

28. Joanne Lynn, "Travels in the Valley of the Shadow," in Howard M. Spiro, Mary G. McCrea Curnen, Enid Peschel, and Deborah St. James, eds., *Empathy and the Practice of Medicine* (New Haven, Conn.: Yale University Press, 1993), p. 52.

29. See, e.g., Lewis Thomas, *The Fragile Species* (New York: Scribner's, 1992), a touching series of reflections that illustrates these points.

30. As a formal discipline, thanatology—the study of dying and of its medical and psychological effects—began in 1967, when Austin H. Kutscher and others established the Foundation of Thanatology at Columbia University. See Nancy Hicks, "Neglect of Dying Patients' Emotional Needs Linked to Cultural Inability to Face Death," *NYT* (26 Aug. 1970): 13.

31. Lisa W. Foderaro, "Death Wishes," *NYT* (3 Apr. 1994): 1.

32. Tom Kuntz, "Death Be Not Unpublishable: The Literature of Good Grief," *NYT* (29 Nov. 1998): 7.

33. Cf. Voltaire's observation: "Man is the only animal that knows he has to die. This is a sad bit of knowledge, but necessary, as long as he is going to have ideas." [*"L'homme est le seul animal qui sache, qu'il doit mourir. Triste connaissance, mais nécessaire puisqu'il a des idées."*] This remark was attributed to Voltaire in Elliott M. Grant, Murray Sachs, and Richard B. Grant, *French Stories, Plays, and Poetry: A First-Year College Reader* (New York: Oxford University Press, 1959), p. 5; no source was given.

34. "The Meaning of Death," *Time* 65, no. 2 (11 Jan.1960): 52, 54.

35. Vincent Mor, David S. Greer, and Robert Kastenbaum, eds., *The Hospice Experiment* (Baltimore: Johns Hopkins University Press, 1988), p. 5.

36. Barney G. Glaser and Anselm L. Strauss, *Awareness of Dying* (Chicago: Aldine Publishing Co., 1965), p. 3.

37. Elisabeth Kübler-Ross, *On Death and Dying* (New York: Macmillan/Collier Books, 1993 [1969]). Among many measures of the book's importance is the reference to its "great success [*grote succes*]" in a book on euthanasia published more than two decades later in Holland. See Gerrit van der Wal, *Euthansie en hulp bij zelfdoding door huisartsen* [*Euthanasia and Suicide with Assistance from Family Doctors*] (Rotterdam: WYT Uitgeefgroep, 1992), p. 132.

38. The stages tend to overlap even for those who do experience them, as Kübler-Ross's chart clearly shows (see Kübler-Ross, *On Death and Dying*, p. 235), but many who can name the stages have ignored that subtlety. The result for some dying persons is more frustration. "All that nonsense that's written about stages of dying," one such patient is quoted as saying, "as if there were complete transitions—rooms that you enter, walk through, then leave behind for good. What rot. The anger, the shock, the unbelievableness, the grief—they are part of each day. And in no particular order, either." Quoting "Gordon," in Arthur Kleinman, *The Illness Narratives: Suffering, Healing, and the Human Condition* (New York: Basic Books, 1988), p. 147.

39. Jessica Mitford, *The American Way of Death* (New York: Simon & Schuster, 1963). The reissuing of the book with some new and updated material thirty-five years later (*The American Way of Death Revisited* [New York: Knopf, 1998]) is further testimony to the book's influence. Like Kübler-Ross's "five stages," Mitford's "American way of death" has become idiomatic.

40. Bert Keizer, *Dancing with Mister D: Notes on Life and Death* (New York: Talese/Doubleday, 1997).

41. Sherwin B. Nuland, *How We Die: Reflections on Life's Final Chapter* (New York: Knopf, 1994).

42. Judy Foreman, "When it is time, there are ways to help death come gently," *BG* (7 Mar. 1994): 29.

43. W. Y. Evans-Wentz, comp. and ed., *The Tibetan Book of the Dead* (New York: Oxford University Press, 1960); also a newer edition, Francesca Fremantle and Chogyam Trungpa, trans./commentator, *The Tibetan Book of the Dead* (Boulder and London: Shambhala, 1975). Tibetan and Buddhist ideas have become available to a wider readership through Lati Rinbochay and Jeffrey Hopkins, *Death, Intermediate State and Rebirth in Tibetan Buddhism* (Valois, N.Y.: Gabriel Press, 1979), and, more recently, Sogyal Rinpoche, *The Tibetan Book of Living and Dying* (San Francisco: HarperSan Francisco, 1992).

44. Inge B. Corless, Barbara B. Germino, and Mary Pittman, eds., *Dying, Death, and Bereavement: Theoretical Perspectives and Other Ways of Knowing* (Boston: Jones and Bartlett, 1994).

45. Examples abound. Among the strengths of physician Timothy E. Quill's *Death and Dignity: Making Choices and Taking Charge* (New York: Norton, 1993) are the cases he describes from his medical practice. Journalist Marilyn Webb, *The Good Death: The New American Search to Reshape the End of Life* (New York: Bantam, 1997), uses both the personal-story and the case-study technique. And one of the

most gripping sections in historian Philippe Ariès's, *The Hour*, is the very personal story of the La Ferronays family in nineteenth-century France (pp. 412–31).

46. For a helpful discussion of the nature of medical knowledge, see Stephen Toulmin, "On the Nature of the Physician's Understanding," *Jrnl. of Phil. and Med.* 1, no. 1 (Mar. 1976): 32–50. See also Samuel Gorovitz and Alasdair MacIntyre, "Toward a Theory of Medical Fallibility," *Jrnl. of Phil. and Med.* 1, no. 1 (Mar. 1976): 51–71; Eric B. Beresford, "Uncertainty and the Shaping of Medical Decisions," *HCR* 21, no. 4 (July-Aug. 1991): 6–11; and John F. Lauerman, "The Elusive Diagnosis," *Harvard Health* (Sept.-Oct. 1997): 19–20, 22. Happily, in an eminently readable recent book by a physician with an intended audience not only of his medical colleagues but also of general readers, the author deals quite concretely with the extent to which medical errors are unavoidable. In part, he argues, this is precisely because of the inherent uncertainty in medical knowledge. See Atul Gawande, *Complications: A Surgeon's Notes on an Imperfect Science* (New York: Metropolitan Books/Henry Holt, 2002).

47. In a remarkably concise fashion, some of this gap is filled by Wanzer, *The End of Life*.

48. Ronald Dworkin, *Life's Dominion: An Argument About Abortion, Euthanasia, and Individual Freedom* (New York: Knopf, 1993), p. 199.

49. According to research conducted by the National Hospice Foundation, however, "Most Americans are completely unaware of hospice services," "Nearly 80 percent of Americans do not think of hospice as a choice for end-of-life care," and "Fewer than 10 percent know that hospice provides pain relief for the terminally ill." See the Web site *http://NHPCO.org* under "Public Engagement Campaign." These statistics are startling.

50. Other organizations besides the National Hospice Organization (since February 2000 known as the National Hospice and Palliative Care Organization [NHPCO]) are working to improve care for dying patients. Many of them adhere to at least some aspects of the Hospice philosophy in what they advocate, as they attempt generally to implement the Hospice approach. In addition to Americans for Better Care of the Dying (ABCD), based at George Washington University's Center to Improve Care of the Dying, there is the Boston-based Institute for Healthcare Improvement (IHI). One proposed "model of care for [the] seriously ill" is "MediCaring," an as-yet-not-implemented idea for "what a revised national vision [of end-of-life care] would look like." The idea is that it "would extend hospice-style symptom management and supportive care to a broader array of individuals and services than is now possible under Medicare." ABCD, *The Advocate's Guide to Better End-of-Life Care: Physician-Assisted Suicide and Other Options* (Washington, D.C.: ABCD, 1997), pp. 73, 56–57, and 75 respectively.

51. ABCD, *Advocate's Guide*, p. 56.

52. "Hospice neither hastens nor postpones death; it affirms life and regards dying as a normal process." From "The Basics of Hospice," a 1996 pamphlet distributed by what was then the National Hospice Organization (NHO).

53. The parallel organization in England is the National Council for Hospice and Specialist Palliative Care Services, Hospice House, 34–44 Britannia Street, London WC1X 9JG.

54. Not everyone who disapproves of the Hemlock/right-to-die approach is necessarily an active supporter of the Hospice approach. Some, like members of

the group Not Dead Yet, (which lobbies for rights for the disabled) appear far more concerned with fighting Hemlock than with supporting Hospice; this particular group was formed with the explicit aim of opposing Jack Kevorkian and "the [unnamed] proponents of assisted suicide for people with disabilities." Fred Pelka, *The Disability Rights Movement* (Santa Barbara, Calif.: ABC-CLIO, 1997), p. 359. A similar stance is taken by The Arc (a national organization on mental retardation). In the summer of 1998, a new "Position Statement" was being circulated among its member-chapters that would make explicit The Arc's "opposition to physician-assisted suicide for people with mental retardation." *The Arc Today* 47, no. 2 (Summer 1998): 1. At the "Decision Making at the End of Life" conference sponsored by the Royal Society of Medicine, which I attended in London, Bert Massie (representing RADAR, an English disability charity) acknowledged that there is very little consensus within the disabled population about appropriate treatment at the end of life, but he nonetheless expressed the standard line of concern that a "right to die" could lead to a "duty to die."

55. I am indebted to physician J. Donald Schultz for this suggestion.

56. Already more than a decade ago the vulnerability of the elderly was seen as a serious problem; see, e.g., Margot Tallmer, Elizabeth R. Prichard, Austin H. Kutscher, et al., eds., *The Life-Threatened Elderly* (New York: Columbia University Press, 1984). More recently—to cite but three examples—are discussions by Denise Niemira, "Life on the Slippery Slope: A Bedside View of Treating Incompetent Elderly Patients," *HCR* 23, no. 3 (May-June 1993): 14–17; Rebecca Dresser and Peter J. Whitehouse, "The Incompetent Patient on the Slippery Slope," *HCR* 24, no. 4 (July-Aug. 1994): 6–12; and Daniel Callahan, "Terminating Life-Sustaining Treatment of the Demented," *HCR* 25, no. 6 (Nov.-Dec. 1995): 25–31.

57. See Timothy E. Quill, Christine Cassel, and Diane E. Meier, "Care of the Hopelessly Ill: Proposed Clinical Criteria for Physician Assisted Suicide," *NEJM* 327, no. 19 (5 Nov. 1992): 1381.

58. Feldman, *Confrontations*, p. 5.

59. Feldman, *Confrontations*, p. 11.

60. See Philippe Ariès, "Part I: Tame Death," *The Hour* (esp. pp. 5–28), as well as "Tamed Death" in his *Western Attitudes toward Death from the Middle Ages to the Present* (Baltimore: Johns Hopkins University Press, 1974), pp. 1–25.

61. Callahan, *Troubled Dream*, p. 30.

62. For a study of this subject (among others), see J. E. Seymour, *Critical Moments: Death and Dying in Intensive Care* (Buckingham, England: Open University Press, 2001). An earlier version of Seymour's Ch. 6 was published earlier as "Negotiating Natural Death in Intensive Care," *Soc. Sci. & Med.* 51, no. 8 (Oct. 2000): 1241–52.

63. See Henry James, *The Wings of the Dove* (Harmondsworth, England: Penguin, 1974 [1902]), p. 369.

64. Another whole area of concern is that of "social death"—frequently though not universally experienced prior to physical death—that may bring with it a period of considerable distress and suffering. The literature on this important topic, which is also one I will not be considering, has enormous range. One good example of work in this field is Helen N. Sweeting and Mary L. M. Gilhooly, "Doctor, Am I Dead? A Review of Social Death in Modern Societies," *Omega: Jrnl. of Death and Dying* 24, no. 4 (1991–92): 251–69.

65. I am indebted to the Rev. James Keck for first suggesting this succinct way of indicating why appeals to religion are problematic when a serious, wholly rational discussion is the object. Philosopher John Rawls makes the same point, more generally: "Where the suppression of liberty is based upon theological principles or matters of faith, no argument is possible." John Rawls, *A Theory of Justice* (Cambridge, Mass.: Harvard University Press, 1971), p. 216.

66. David A. Asch, John Hansen-Flaschen, and Paul N. Lanken, "Decisions to Limit or Continue Life-sustaining Treatment by Critical Care Physicians in the United States: Conflicts Between Physicians' Practices and Patients' Wishes," *Am. Jrnl. of Resp. and Crit. Care Med.* 151 (1995): 289.

67. Stuart J. Youngner, "Futility in Context," *JAMA* 264, no. 10 (12 Sept. 1990): 1295.

68. John Saunders, "Medical Futility: CPR," in Robert Lee and Derek Morgan, eds., *Death Rites: Law and Ethics at the End of Life* (London: Routledge, 1994), p. 85.

69. J. Chris Hackler and F. Charles Hiller, "Family Consent to Orders Not to Resuscitate: Reconsidering Hospital Policy," *JAMA* 264, no. 10 (12 Sept. 1990): 1282.

70. Emma J. Aarons and Nicholas J. Beeching, "Survey of 'Do not resuscitate' orders in a district general hospital," *BMJ* 303 (14 Dec. 1991): 1504.

71. Lawrence J. Schneiderman, Nancy S. Jecker, and Albert R. Jonsen, "Medical Futility: Its Meaning and Ethical Implications," *Ann. Int. Med.* 112, no. 12 (15 June 1990): 953. Two letters and a response from the authors appeared two issues later, *Ann. Int. Med.* 114, no. 2 (15 Jan. 1991): 169–70. Daniel Callahan reviews and evaluates some of the work on "futility"—including this last-named article—in his "Medical Futility, Medical Necessity: The Problem-Without-A-Name," *HCR* 21, no. 4 (July-Aug. 1991): 30–35.

72. Nancy S. Jecker, "Futile Treatment and the Ethics of Medicine," *Report for the Institute for Philosophy & Policy* (School of Public Affairs, University of Maryland) 15, no. 1 (Winter 1995): 11.

73. J. Saunders, "Medical Futility," in Lee and Morgan, eds., *Death Rites,* p. 85.

2

Origins of the Debate

We talked together with Life, but Death broke in . . .
——Merrill Moore[1]

Understanding the history of the Hospice and Hemlock movements should make it easier to grasp how we find ourselves where we are today with respect to death and dying. A good historical backdrop will prove helpful when we put on center stage such crucial contemporary issues as whether there is a "right to die" (Chapter 3) and the significance of the legal status of euthanasia in the Netherlands for us in the United States (Chapter 4). First, a few reflections on the history of doctors and death will enable us to put the origins and roles of the two movements in context.

The advent of "miracle drugs" in the 1930s, followed by more recent applications of technology to medicine, made it suddenly seem that doctors could stop death in its tracks. Unfortunately, once it was seen that death still would not be stayed, too many physicians tended to withdraw. When the patient really was dying, someone else (nursing staff, family, friends) had to take over. As a result, dying patients commonly complain that they feel abandoned by their doctors. We have allowed doctors to step off stage, to move into the wings.

In earlier periods, that would have been all right. Doctors played little or no role at the bedside of the dying patient; death has only relatively recently been medicalized. Originally an event for family and friends, open and public, death was unattended by professionals. Later, when they were present at the deathbed, it was priests and other religious figures rather than physicians who were typically the first to be called as death approached. Only since the eighteenth century has the world of medicine with increasing regularity "control[led] and administer[ed] the actual process of dying."[2] Even then, few people died from lengthy illnesses, so there was little warrant for seeking a physician's help. In the nineteenth century, infectious and communicable diseases, poor nutrition, and personal hygiene that left much to be desired constituted the major health problems in the United States. These issues continued well into the twentieth century.[3]

In a time when most people died young—of accidents or of acute childhood diseases—physicians were as powerless as the parents and other loved ones who surrounded the dying. Prior to our current, post-antibiotic age of dying, the crucial issue for many was whether there would be sufficient warning to go through the necessary rituals when Death (usually personified) approached. In the early medieval period, death was considered a benign event, "tame" (to use Philippe Ariès's evocative descriptor[4]). Dying then was a set piece of what we would call "performance art" today.[5] "Knowing that his end was near," Ariès tells us, "the dying person prepared for death." He goes on to say that "death was a ritual organized by the dying person himself, who presided over it and knew its protocol."[6]

Today, finally, people just do live longer. Chronic diseases of middle and old age (such as heart disease, cancer, and stroke) consume much of the time and energy of those in the health-care business and lead in many cases to "more lonely death in old age."[7] The modern-day alienation from death and its rituals, it has been claimed, stems in part from the way we as a society have abrogated our responsibilities, allowing "specialists" (physicians, nurses, and technicians) to take over.[8]

Ariès's account of our changing attitudes toward death makes vivid how small a part doctors used to play. If a doctor was summoned at all near the hour of death, it was not because anyone expected medical miracles, for "miracles" were understood to be divine in origin and not to have anything to do with the meager skills of the medical profession. Rather, the doctor, simply by virtue of being a member of one of the professions, played a special ceremonial role much like that of the priest. Just as priests were thought to have some healing powers—a return to or remnant of the belief in classical Greece that gods (Apollo, and later his son Asclepius) were the source of healing—doctors were thought to have quasi-priestly powers.[9] Such was the potency of the professions. Dying was tame, dying was public, dying was a ceremony to be ritually celebrated (whether by doctors or by priests was not important).

Then, late in the nineteenth century, a revolution in attitude began. Death began to be seen as something shameful, messy, dirty—something that needed to be kept hidden, private. And one way to do this was, for the first time really, to actively involve doctors. Let them deal with the dying, let them take the dying out of their homes and put them in hospitals, where death could be (perhaps) cleaned up and (increasingly, in the twentieth century) reduced to a technical phenomenon. Death was no longer a personal or a public event, but a medical problem for doctors to handle.[10] Doctors began to be called to the deathbed, often to the exclusion of priests; it was the physicians who came to be revered as high priests in white coats with special powers.

Exactly what is expected of the doctors standing at the side of the deathbed has also changed considerably through the centuries, however, as have most other aspects of the doctor-patient relationship. What is considered appropriate behavior for physicians when their patients are dying continues to evolve. The implications of innovations in the practice of medicine as well as in the way doctors and the dying interact (despite or because of new protocols) and what role tradition should play are still neither well understood nor agreed upon. One thing is clear. In the United States (though not only here), the basis for doctors' attitudes toward how they should treat their dying patients has long been found in the principle of *primum non nocere* (first, do not harm) passed down from Hippocrates, as we will see. But alongside that principle, the huge array of medical means available today for doing positive *good* has effected a shift in emphasis. Medical schools stress that the doctor's job is to cure patients, and we as a society re-inforce that by first marveling at and then expecting miracle cures at every turn. The death of a patient begins to look and feel like medical failure; the so-called technological imperative (if it can be done, it will be—or should be—done) takes over. Increasingly, we focus on encouraging physicians less to avoid harm than to do as much good as they can. Death is no longer seen as an unavoidable and wholly natural biological event, but as a "harm." As such, it is something doctors want as little to do with as possible.

Jean Berger, the author of *A Fortunate Man* (1967) (about a Scottish country doctor), therefore sounds rather old fashioned when he writes that the "doctor is the familiar of death. When we call for a doctor, we are asking him to cure us and to relieve our suffering, but, if he cannot cure us, we are also asking him to witness our dying. The value of the witness is that he has seen so many others die."[11] Too often, we draw a distinction between "curing" and that next stage of "witnessing" (usually included under the rubric of "caring")—as if doctors were not supposed to be involved in both. Why the separation? Why the division between "curing" and "caring"? Doctors surely should not be able altogether to escape an intimate connection with death.

What "curing" and "caring" have to do with each other—particularly at that all-important point when what might count as "curing" is impossible and perhaps no longer even desirable—is central to this whole study. Before looking at the history of the modern Hospice movement (including its older roots) and the even newer Hemlock (right-to-die) movement, however, we need to return for a moment to the beginnings of Western civilization. For it is there, as already hinted, that we find the foundation of present-day attitudes toward the question of how doctors should treat their dying patients.

STARTING WITH HIPPOCRATES

Over and above the generalized precept of *primum non nocere,* credited to the ancient Greek physician Hippocrates, the most commonly cited traditional statement of what physicians should (or, more precisely, should not) do with and for their dying patients comes from the so-called Hippocratic Oath.[12] This Oath is part of a wide range of documents that, taken together, have come to be called the "Hippocratic Corpus." Today it is generally understood that the sixty or so treatises that comprise the Corpus—all of them anonymous, most though not all of them written between 430 and 330 B.C.—are the product of numerous medical writers, "belonging to different groups or schools and representing in many cases quite opposed viewpoints."[13] No one has yet established definitively which treatises are actually the work of Hippocrates. Nevertheless, "Hippocrates still represents an ethical ideal, the ideal of the compassionate, discreet and selfless doctor."[14] This, despite the fact that we know very little about the man himself, and despite the fact that historians now understand much of his reputation to have been the result of latter-day attempts to ground practice in ancient authority.[15]

Hence it may be that Hippocrates himself neither wrote nor ever spoke the words of the Oath that bears his name.[16] Authorship apart, however, "the ethical content is largely consistent with the genuine Hippocratic writings." Few doctors today would deny (though they might want to argue about details) that "the ethical precepts of the oath remain the basis for all later discussions of those moral considerations which must guide the physician."[17]

For present purposes, the most important passage in the Oath is the line "I will not give a fatal draught to anyone if I am asked, nor will I suggest any such thing."[18] Yet those who quote this passage do not bother to explain why this precept should be rigidly followed while some of the others in the Oath can be ignored (such as the promise to teach the "science [of medicine]" to all the sons of one's own teacher without charging any fee). Similarly, those who are quick to insist on the enduring legitimacy of giving no "fatal draught to anyone" rarely have much to say about why the physician should never—as the same passage continues—"cut, not even for stone" (that is, never engage in even minor surgery). In other words, the historic model tends to be called upon when it is useful and dismissed when it is not.

The implied Hippocratic injunction against physicians doing anything that could be construed as actively assisting their patients to die has carried enormous moral weight among physicians in the Western tradition for centuries. Three decades ago, an editorial in the *Journal of the American Medical Association* (*JAMA*) bemoaned that "the ceremonial administration of the oath to medical students seems, lamentably, to be declining."[19] In 1989, however, all the accredited medical schools in the United States used an oath as part of their graduation ceremonies (some gave students a choice of oaths); sixty of the oaths (fewer than half those used) had wording that at least resembled the text of the Hippocratic Oath. Although there is considerable overlap in what students swear to in these different oaths, only about half explicitly invoke the principle of non-maleficence; a full two-thirds, in contrast, mention beneficence. This tilt toward the positive virtue of doing good and the lesser emphasis on avoiding harm is interesting, and perhaps important—but it does not bespeak a weakening of the powerful tradition of the Hippocratic Oath. Both principles are involved there.[20]

Furthermore, the variations in wording do nothing to settle the issue of whether helping a patient die counts as a harm or a benefit. This, then, is our starting point. Hippocrates—that traditional paragon of medical ethics, famous among other things for insisting on thoughtful and compassionate care of patients[21]—seems to be saying doctors must not aid their patients in their dying. Because the prohibition of the "fatal draught" is so explicit, the burden of proof has long been thought to rest on those who think (or want to argue) that, at least under some conditions, it might be appropriate for physicians directly to help their patients die, perhaps indeed going so far as to recommend (or even to offer) a "fatal draught." On the other side of the fence, the Hippocratic injunction (and its parallel in other oaths) has given secular support to those who for largely religious reasons believe that human beings have no right to dispose of what God has granted (that is, their life). The questions that arise are these: How literally is the prohibition of a "fatal draught" to be taken? Is "Don't assist in a patient's suicide" what the author of the Oath was really saying, and is it what he would say today? Even if it is and he would, are there contemporary arguments that permit overriding this traditional position? Are any compromises possible that will make way for a middle ground?

Just as it has long been understood that medicine in the classical period cannot fairly be judged solely by modern standards, so twenty-first-century medicine cannot reasonably rely solely on teachings of the classical period. In particular, one must be careful about picking and choosing only the parts one likes of a text like the Hippocratic Oath. If only some precepts laid down by Hippocrates and his followers are to be followed today, we need solid reasons both for the discarding and for the retaining. We cannot, however, escape the fact that the oft-repeated Hippocratic

injunction against giving patients "a fatal draught" remains the underlying principle of much current thinking about medical care of the dying.

HOSPICE

"Hospice care" as a concept and even the word "hospice" itself have
fairly recently become part of common parlance, but neither the word nor
the concept is really new. The emergence of the modern Hospice movement, modeled on but different from its antecedents in the Middle Ages,
has had a dramatic (and largely positive) effect on contemporary attitudes
toward death and dying. The origins of the movement and the ideas behind it will help us understand "Hospice" (with capital "H") and how to
distinguish it from "hospice care" (with lower-case "h").

The etymology of "hospice" shows that the Latin word *hospes*, curiously
enough, meant both "host" and "guest"—thus tying inextricably together
the role of the carer and the cared-for. *Hospes* evolved into *hospitium* (from
which we get "hospitable," for instance) as well as French *hôpital* (whence
"hospital") and *hôtel-Dieu* (thence English "hostel" and "hotel"). Today,
though hotels and hospitals still share some features, the two institutions
are so far removed from each other in most important ways that it is easy
to forget their common origin. Yet there are similarities, crucial to the
modern hospice, as has been pointed out: Each is "a place of meeting, a
way station, a place of transit, of arrival and departure."[22]

In the Middle Ages, hospices—"a blend of guest house and infirmary
where all comers were given food, shelter, and care until they died or set
out again, refreshed and renewed, on their journeys"—were scattered
across Europe. They were "a manifestation of a sacred worldview that led
monks and nuns to act out of the belief that service to one's neighbor is a
sign of love and dedication to God."[23] Today the best known of these hospices are probably those founded during the Crusades, like the Knights
Hospitaller of the Order of St. John in Jerusalem. Yet long before the medieval period, there were hospices already in the ancient world.[24]

Anyone who has arrived in an unfamiliar town feeling ill, or who has
failed to find a satisfactory place to lay a weary head after walking (or
even driving) many miles, can easily understand the appeal of such foundations. Pilgrims to the Ganges, in ancient India, found facilities where
they could die (after which their ashes would be scattered in the sacred
river, which was the point of the pilgrimage). The ancient Greeks and
Romans both built facilities to care for strangers, sick or transient. Later,
Christians and Moslems alike viewed caring for the sick as a religious
duty; the result was that many hospices were founded all across Europe
and Asia Minor. Accepting the responsibility for the "care of strangers,"
whether religiously motivated or not, is characteristic of the movement
to develop hospitals (and related facilities) in general.[25]

Hospices did not initially specialize in care for the dying (the Indian example mentioned above is an exception). The emphasis was rather simply on offering assistance to the sick, the indigent, or the weary traveler. For Christians in particular, working in a hospice provided an opportunity for sacrifice in the service of others in this life that was especially appealing; it was a way to find favor in the next life. If those being cared for could be helped in their own preparation for death, so much the better.

With the rise of early modern medicine and the accompanying formation of a secular medical profession, control of health care began to slip away from the Church. In England, for instance, care of the indigent fell in the first instance to towns, leading to the creation of almshouses and workhouses to accommodate "the chronically ill, poor, or dying who were unwelcome in hospitals." Doctors were sometimes called to tend the workhouse residents.[26] Accommodations in these establishments were often so inadequate that by the late nineteenth century it was clear there was a need once again for the old traditional hospices. Many hospices had been converted to hospitals, with all the changes in character that our use of those words today would lead us to expect.

The Church was also by no means out of the health-care business. An 1879 foundation in Ireland appears to be the first established explicitly for the purpose of giving palliative care to the dying. Others soon followed, including St. Luke's House of the Dying Poor in Bayswater (1893) and St. Joseph's in London (1905), both of which would play roles roughly a half century later in the establishment of the modern Hospice movement. All of these institutions were affiliated one way or another with Catholic or Anglican religious orders or were under the direction of one or another of the Protestant denominations.

Today, "hospice" stands first and foremost for an approach to the treatment of dying patients (not necessarily a religiously grounded approach) that emphasizes "comfort care." The basic idea is that palliative care (defined as, for example, "symptom control, effective communication and measures to support the quality of life for a dying person and their family"[27]) and individualized treatment plans are offered on a continuing basis, and aggressively, to all dying patients. Such care is viewed as especially important at the point when "cure" is no longer possible.

Most commentators give credit for founding the modern Hospice movement to Dame Cicely Saunders.[28] But the idea of hospices did not spring full-grown from her brow—as she herself has repeatedly acknowledged—and there is still a need to distinguish between the specific ideology of Hospice and the more general idea of hospice care, as we shall shortly see. The story of how Saunders came to devote her professional life to the care of dying patients has often been told, though usually in quite fragmentary fashion, by Saunders herself[29] and by others,[30] but a bit of background is appropriate here.

At St. Luke's, where Saunders worked as a volunteer before going to medical school, she for the first time experienced an institution aimed specifically at caring for the dying. At St. Joseph's (where she held her first post as medical officer), she saw for herself and had an opportunity to demonstrate to others what a difference adequate pain control could make in the lives of dying patients. Indeed, it was at St. Joseph's that the seed for St. Christopher's Hospice in the London suburb of Sydenham was planted. (Though St. Christopher's is regularly referred to as if it were the home base of the Hospice movement, it is not and never was an official "movement headquarters.") "Without this opportunity [at St. Joseph's]," Dame Cicely has said, "I do not think the modern hospice movement would have been established and I am everlastingly grateful to the patients and Sisters of St. Joseph's, who, together with David Tasma [one of Dr. Saunders's dying patients, whom she credits with having 'sparked the inspiration for hospice'] and the patients of St. Luke's, I see as the true founders."[31]

When St. Christopher's was established in 1967, it was clear that it was to be a "Christian as well as a medical foundation."[32] That was partly as a result of Saunders's own motivation ("I saw this as a vocation from God"; "I believed so firmly that this was God's plan"[33]). But it is also true that the new establishment was a direct descendant of then-existing facilities run under Christian direction providing institutional care for the terminally ill.

At least one observer has claimed that the "modern hospice movement saw itself as new and unique," committed among other things to permanently altering a landscape littered with "health care practices that dehumanized or ignored the dying person." Some of the "religious devotees" at facilities where the dying were treated, though sympathetic to the practices of the new movement, were nonetheless "uninterested in the political struggles." In the end, it may be that the respective missions of the older hospices and of the new ones—at least in the United States—are not identical. One aims at caring; the other is determined also to reform medical care. Hospice work in any case "provided something different."[34] In both the United States and England, the literature on hospice care, though replete with references to "the modern Hospice Movement" (thus acknowledging predecessors), makes it sound as if what we now have is a wholly new endeavor.

Exactly what hospice care is and does cannot easily be presented in a short space, not least because there are, in literature on the subject (including more-or-less official publications of the Hospice movement), "various definitions of the essential characteristics of hospice."[35] The National Hospice Organization (NHO) in the United States put it this way a few years back: "A hospice is a program of palliative and supportive services which provides physical, psychological, social and spiritual care for dying

persons and their families."[36] In 2001, the Web page giving general information about the renamed organization (National Hospice and Palliative
Care Organization [NHPCO]) words it slightly differently: "Considered
to be the model for quality, compassionate care at the end of life, hospice
care involves a team-oriented approach of expert medical care, pain management, and emotional and spiritual support expressly tailored to the
patient's wishes. Emotional and spiritual support also is extended to the
family and loved ones."[37] The change in wording from "program" to "approach" is appropriate and results in a more accurate statement. "The bare
outlines of the hospice approach were encapsulated in recommendations
made by an international task force in 1975," we are told. The "two very
basic guidelines for care" that came out of this work were as follows: "(1)
the terminally ill person's own preferences and life-style must be taken
into account in all decision making; and (2) family members and other
caregivers also have legitimate needs and interests that must be taken into
consideration."[38]

Perhaps the most telling feature of talk about hospice is how frequently
words like "experiment," "alternative," and "better" come into play
(prime examples appear in the titles of books I have been citing and quoting). Hospice is seen to represent not only a different but an improved way
of coping with the dying process. Care in hospices aims to assure that no
one dies alone or in pain. Longtime Hospice physician Joanne Lynn was
quoted just prior to the oral argument before the Supreme Court in two
"right to die" cases, *Washington et al. v. Glucksberg* and *Vacco v. Quill*,[39] saying "[n]o one needs to be alone or in pain."[40] Ira Byock (also a physician),
president of the Academy of Hospice and Palliative Medicine, stresses
these aspects of the classic Hospice position in the introduction to his
book, *Dying Well*: "I think it is realistic to hope for a future in which nobody has to die alone and nobody has to die with their pain untreated."[41]

Hospice emphasizes the support and simple presence that family and
friends can offer dying persons, and pain management—"the most important form of palliative care that hospices provide."[42] This translates into
a thoroughgoing team approach to care for the dying as well as a focus
on the needs of the patient's principal caregivers; it translates further into
an aggressive and sometimes creative use of symptom management and
pain control.[43] The result (insist most Hospice apologists) is that, because
"Hospice affirms life,"[44] hospice patients are given the opportunity to "live
fully until they die."[45] This is the underlying theme of many articles about
Hospice, in England as well as in the United States.[46] Hospice is thus not
a place, but—according to Dame Cicely herself—a matter of "attitudes and
skills and a philosophy."[47]

And yet, of course, at least some features of that "philosophy," and the
"attitudes and skills," are not necessarily restricted to those who work
within Hospice—by which I mean within or for an organization that

belongs, in the United States, to the NHPCO. The primary difference between those engaged in "hospice care" outside the movement and those inside is apt to be the degree to which they accept the entire ideology of the movement. The insistence that no one need die alone or in pain, the emphasis on the need to take a terminally ill person's own preferences and lifestyle into account in all decision making, and the effort to include consideration for family members' and other caregivers' legitimate needs and interests are all things with which anyone engaged in hospice care is likely to be comfortable. In addition, however, there is an underlying mantra (what Cicely Saunders means by the "philosophy") that is basic to the Hospice movement: Nothing is to be done that would either prolong life artificially or hasten the dying process unnaturally. This is the central, ideological basis of Hospice (though there is evidence that not everyone within Hospice is able fully to support it).

The differences are likely to be noticed only at the very end of a patient's life. The support given patient and family alike, coupled with the aggressive pursuit of palliation for those in pain, is something on which all hospice workers agree. That this kind of care is important and startlingly new, not something that can be taken for granted in our current medico-technological climate, is confirmed by too many tales of distress at a bitterly won release from death. Most of us have heard about or witnessed such deaths. But new efforts are being made, according to a December 2000 *New York Times* article. Some hospitals were said to "have changed the medications they use, adding newer pain medications and interventions . . . ; combining pain medications; and decreasing the use of drugs . . . [that have] adverse effects on the central nervous system."[48] And in 2001, "new standards from the Joint Commission on Accreditation of Healthcare Organizations require health-care facilities to assess and manage pain."[49]

The idea that Hospice involves something new and different is given credence by stories Hospice caregivers themselves tell. Joanne Lynn's essay, "Travels in the Valley of the Shadow," is a case in point. There she recounts her "extraordinary good fortune [in having] to take an undervalued and academically meaningless job . . . [in] a nascent hospice program." Instead of finding the work depressing, she found it supremely rewarding. When a dying patient "had so many good times in our care," and when the family could look back on "the good time that they shared under the shadow of death," Lynn insists, the caregivers "can be confident that lives were made better by their efforts. What more," she adds rhetorically, "can we ask of our work?"[50] Anyone reading Sandol Stoddard's *Hospice Movement* (1992 [1978]) and Anne Munley's *Hospice Alternative* (1983), with their often-detailed accounts of cases in one hospice or another, is also likely to come away inspired. Working with the dying, at least the Hospice way, is typically seen as an uplifting way to help people "live fully while they are dying."

These same books, again because of the myriad personal stories, give as good an idea as one could hope for (apart from direct experience) of what living and dying under Hospice care is like. Throughout, a refreshing emphasis is laid on the attention paid to each patient's individual needs. One important aspect of the method by which this is accomplished is the multi-professional team that, among other things, is expected "to listen to and care for the whole person."[51] Moreover, care is personalized in every sense of the word. In addition to the pain control that is paramount in Hospice philosophy ("[s]ometimes rather sophisticated medications are necessary"), Hospice caregivers are trained to follow procedures for relief of other kinds of distress, some of which "can be surprisingly simple. Gentle massage, a soft pillow placed just so, a subtle change in diet, a tempting drink, or time taken simply to be present, quietly caring and listening, recognizing the person as a unique and valued individual—these things can truly heal the dying, even when cure has become impossible."[52]

Such language is typical of Hospice literature; it reflects also an observation attributed to Cicely Saunders that "[h]ealing a person does not always mean curing a disease."[53] Joanne Lynn, likewise, tells a story of a patient for whom "profound suffering" had such personal, redemptive significance that the pain was "not an appropriate target for treatment."[54] A willingness to respect such an attitude is difficult to imagine in a traditional hospital setting. There, the medical personnel are still generally presumed to know what is best for the patient and no one is likely to think pain should be ignored, even if it is often not aggressively treated. (But even under hospice care such requests for non-treatment are not always respected. Stories exist of Hospice patients who, for their own psychological or other reasons, have *not* wanted heavy doses of morphine and have had to argue with Hospice nurses who "knew" what should be done.[55])

Perhaps as good an indication as there is of the powerfully positive effect exposure to Hospice care can have appears in Greg Palmer's somewhat eccentric discussion of death, which he sardonically refers to as the "Trip of a Lifetime":

[W]atching hospices in action, seeing what Sacred Heart in Sydney did for Ian, what Evergreen did for Ed and Anne, it's hard not to sound like the chief lobbyist for the Amalgamated Association of Hospices. When I walked into the lobby of Evergreen once, it didn't smell like a hospital or death, it smelled like lasagna. Volunteer Jane Quirck has a great lasagna recipe and frequently mixes up a batch in the family kitchen. Given the choice, who wouldn't want to die in a place that smelled like lasagna?[56]

The point being made here is independent of what is being stressed when the mantra about not prolonging life or hastening death is repeated. It is the nature of the care, not necessarily the Hospice movement, that determines whether there shall be lasagna.

As already mentioned, some commentators have argued that the Hospice movement is above all political, an endeavor aimed at reforming medicine from the inside out.[57] Saunders's account of her own professional development supports this position. Still, just how successful the reforming process has been remains an open question; the influence has undoubtedly been considerable, though nowhere nearly so widespread as one might have wished. Siebold devotes an entire chapter to "The Movement's Accomplishments,"[58] claiming that the greatest impetus for the creation of programs to respond to the needs of the terminally ill have come from St. Christopher's and "Cicely Saunders's modern hospice concept." She also argues, however, that the Hospice movement "might have better managed [its] political course."[59]

Writer and sociologist Tony Walter (in England), while acknowledging that "hospices were founded rapidly in the United States once federal reimbursement from Medicare" came into play, argues that the Hospice movement "has not transferred well . . . to other European nations." In addition, he is at pains to point out that "[o]nly a small minority of people die in or are cared for by hospices," though he goes on to credit hospices (and thus the Hospice movement) as the "major promoters of the idea that patients should die as they choose."[60] This is a more complicated political issue than sometimes seems to have been recognized by those within Hospice; what they mean by letting patients "die as they choose" is not what the right-to-die (Hemlock) supporters mean, as we shall see. Walter's observation evokes the important issue of how much control dying patients ought to have over their own dying—an issue that is by no means unique to supporters of Hospice or purveyors of hospice care outside the movement, let alone to Hemlock supporters.

Certainly Joanne Lynn makes clear, in the essay of hers quoted earlier, that she sees the need to change the standard of care for such patients as a political issue: "Responsibility for the care of patients cannot end with the care of each patient. Each of us who participate[s] in this endeavor also bear some responsibility for sustaining and improving a system of care so that it regularly and readily provides optimal care." And that means for all citizens. The Medicare "hospice benefit" (added in 1982) is not so fair or far-reaching as it needs to be, for "the entire issue of eligibility turns on [a] definition [that makes] very few eligible. . . . So, our major national commitment to improved care of the dying [which Lynn identifies with Hospice], turns out to be available, with only a little overstatement, only to those who have homes, families, some wealth, and convenient diagnoses."[61] Another researcher into how non-medical factors affect end-of-life care says that despite "continual increases in use of the benefit, there also have been persistent concerns that many people who could benefit from hospice care do not receive it."[62] In light of this strongly worded sentiment, it is not surprising that Lynn, now at The Center to Improve Care of the Dying (at George Washington University), has spearheaded a new organization: Americans for Better Care of the Dying (ABCD).[63] "[D]edicated to public information and policy advocacy to improve the last phase of life," the organization is too new for its long-term effectiveness to be judged. But that it has a political agenda of major importance is evident.[64] This is not quite the same as saying that Hospice is a political movement, but the overtones are there—and the casts of characters have considerable overlap. Lynn herself has had years of experience in hospice care, much though not all of it within the Hospice movement. She has issued an explicit challenge to any who will listen: "We must also dedicate substantial effort to reforming the health care system so that everyone can expect to live well as they pass through the valley of the shadow of death."[65]

The growth and spread of the Hospice movement has occurred, it is clear, in tandem with a great upsurge of interest in palliative care. A recent book evaluating palliative care makes frequent reference to "palliative care specialists"—meaning those (nurses and physicians alike) who are engaged in palliative care with the benefit of some degree of "specialist training."[66] Clearly palliative care has marched forward not only under the banner of Hospice. Despite the importance of its role, Hospice cannot claim all the credit for the improvements in this area. As we will see, some of the more explicitly socio-political and legal discussions and activities around death and dying in recent years have helped dramatically improve care for dying patients.

Not very many people in this country (either in- or outside mainstream health-care organizations) took much notice of the new movement until 1971, when the first Hospice unit in the United States was established in Connecticut and began offering specialized home-care services for dying patients.[67] Depending on how the figures are interpreted, the growth of the movement in this country since then has been rapid[68]—or distressingly slow. The latter view is taken by those who look at the immense need; the number of presumably dying patients being more or less warehoused in nursing homes or other long-term-care facilities in this country far outstrips the number of available Hospice beds. Among those surveying the larger landscape is pain-management expert Kathleen Foley, who observed in 1997 that "about 1.6 million dying people a year would be good candidates for hospice care but that only about 350,000 get it."[69]

Yet this may be an unnecessarily gloomy view.[70] Increasingly, when mention is made of someone's impending death, the topic of hospice care is raised (whether hopefully or despairingly is a separate matter[71]). In other words, though there are not enough beds available for all those who could benefit from hospice care, it is nonetheless the case that the word "hospice" tends to come into play when someone is known to be dying. More and more people know about the theoretical possibility of hospice care, and the initial assumption is that this is the kind of care they believe they want for themselves or their loved ones when they are dying. No doubt the frequency with which "hospice" is mentioned in the media is part of the story.[72] The situation is improving; today it is no longer necessary for Cicely Saunders to come to this country to help with the formation of a new hospice unit, as she did when the first one in Connecticut was being formed. We have models aplenty, even if what they are and do still needs explanation.

Less understood than Hospice is what palliative care more generally can offer patients. Specialists in Hospice and Palliative Care Medicine (a new specialty in the United States—the American Board for this subspecialty was not established until the mid-1990s) know they need to spell out even the most basic information. In England, Australia, and several other countries, palliative care is today a medical discipline with "standing like any other specialty." The development has been slower in the United States, though there are now more than 800 Board-certified palliative care specialists in this country.[73]

We have, however, a very long way to go before this most desired of all the benefits of hospice care has become routine and available to all. We need doctors (in and out of Hospice) to direct their classic willingness to "do everything possible" for their patients on different features of intensive care than that expression usually conjures up. Rather than focusing on the possible benefits of dramatic procedures or tricky surgery, rather than imposing still further medications on their dying patients or routinely using CPR when a patient stops breathing, doctors need to be willing to engage equally boldly in pain control. We need heroic measures, but not of the desperate, last-minute, "this just might work" technological variety. The heroism called for does not entail being particularly selfless or brave; what is needed is a heroism that truly centers on the patient's best interests, on care rather than cure. We need more heroic efforts, for example, to reduce or even eliminate pain. Until doctors engage more vigorously in practices aimed at palliation, dying patients are likely to look elsewhere for help.

But where we go from here is less clear. A "hospice benefit" is increasingly included in health insurance plans and is available through Medicare,[74] but Joanne Lynn's somewhat depressing account makes clear how unfairly it actually works. On the other hand, as palliative care itself becomes a better-established area of specialization for physicians (there are only nineteen palliative care fellowship programs in the country, according to Foley, now director of the Open Society Institute's Project on Death in America[75]), the goals of Hospice—that no one should have to die alone or in pain—are likely to be met with increasing frequency.

Still, the details of how these goals are to be reached have yet to be worked out. There is currently little reason to think we have progressed much beyond where we were in 1992, when the following challenge was issued: "What remains undefined is the construction of death in our culture. Is dying a medical event or an event in the life cycle?"[76] Yet it seems unlikely that hospice care will turn out to have been nothing more than a passing fad, given the improvements we have seen and the interest many in the media have taken in issues connected with death and dying. Hospice does seem destined to join the list of movements that have "changed the conversation," as newspaperman David M. Shribman once put it.[77]

Until each of us individually decides the question for ourselves how to "construct" death, we are not in a good position to answer questions about our own deaths. Is death a medical event to be managed technologically, or is it a life-cycle event through which humane and compassionate caregivers can help each of us pass? Also, the physician—for better, for worse—is still the primary figure (other than the dying person), and so we need also to be able to articulate what we think the physician's role should be in each individual case. When we can do that, we may be able to give a more general policy answer to the question of what it is appropriate for dying patients to expect from their physicians by way of assistance.

Is there a downside to the Hospice movement or to hospice care? The question is an important one, and, superficially, the answer seems easy. But it is an answer with two parts. Any institution that improves care for the dying is a good thing. Yet any institution or organization run by human beings is bound to have its weaknesses. Certainly when what is at issue is something as complex, serious, and varied as how to treat a stunning array of human beings as they face the end of life, there are bound to be situations where Hospice works less satisfactorily than others. One problem, namely the lack of access (for any one of several different reasons), has already been touched upon. Absence of agreement about when it is appropriate to initiate hospice care is another critical issue. But there are as well more subtle and controversial concerns, which have also been alluded to in the discussion above. One is that "Hospice" has become associated with death and dying to an extent that makes some people reject hospice care at a point when they could benefit from it. Accepting hospice care sounds to many like the first tolling of the death knell. "The very name hospice is frightening," one writer points out. "It may mean 'good death' to health care workers and the healthy, but the operative word is 'death' for the terminal."[78]

Also, in the minds of many, Hospice advocates and workers are vulnerable to the criticism that they have too rigid a view of how people should die. There is, one student of the subject argues, "a contradiction within hospices. On the one hand they are committed to letting patients live as they wish until they die. On the other hand, hospices have a very clear idea of 'the good death' as one in which patient and family accept the terminal diagnosis and in which the actual death is peaceful and preferably in the patient's own home."[79] In another study, designed to explore whether institutionalizing hospice care is likely to compromise the movement's founding ideals, the authors found that there does seem to be a form of "good death" that is recognized as something like the Hospice movement way of dying. There tends to be an approved "Hospice Story" of how to die that "potentially implies rigidity of definitions and limitations to spontaneity." The "Good Death" experience is told and retold, and "becomes what is expected and usual; it becomes routinized and objectified, acting as a symbolic vehicle and guide to future action. . . . These events become ritualized; rhetoric and powerful imagery work to reinforce shared meaning."[80]

Corroboration for the accuracy of this analysis is easy to find. In a passage that fairly cries out "just come watch us at work and you'll see how beautiful what we do is," Anne Munley writes that "[j]udgments about such care cannot be made in the abstract but must be grounded in concrete detail, in the experience of those who have participated in a hospice program. By entering into their world and attempting to see, hear, think, and feel hospice as they do, one can begin to comprehend the significance of the hospice approach." She quotes a patient's blunt comparison of acute-care hospitals and hospices: "'Hospice cares for the patient for the patient's good. The hospital cares for the patient for the hospital's good.'"[81] Yet patients who do not meet the Hospice's criteria determining who should be given terminal sedation, for example, may have to suffer even though they are in great pain and are very ready to die. Timothy Quill relates seeing such a case on a visit to St. Christopher's itself. The first patient he saw there was a woman who was "very, very, very sick and very ready to die"; the experience, as might be expected, colored his view of Hospice care St. Christopher's-style.[82]

We also see the hint of a problem in the negative reactions of several college students when the executive director of a local hospice addressed their class. They seem to have found her explanation of Hospice policies and practices self-satisfied or self-righteous. No doubt their responses were as much a reflection of the 20-somethings' disinclination to be told what to do by anyone as it was a reaction to the rigidity of Hospice as outlined by this particular Hospice advocate.[83] Those same students might have come away with a very different impression of Hospice if they had been exposed to the views of the executive director and other workers and volunteers at a different Hospice. There the staff expressed such a wide range of views on what was acceptable in care for the dying that it was difficult to credit the charges of doctrinaire or rigid attitudes sometimes leveled at Hospice supporters.[84] What we see, then, are that individuals working within the "system" can maintain the individuality of their responses to death and dying even as they publicly pledge allegiance to the Hospice movement and its ideology. But just as clearly, some caregivers within Hospice do have a strong ideological basis for doing the work they do, and they often find it difficult to relax their standards when faced with dying persons who do not agree with their ideology.[85]

Finally, some people argue there is a tendency within the Hospice movement to rely on the emotional power of the movement's claims to make points, with no serious effort to produce supporting arguments. The result is a set of "mantras," which initially sound like straightforward and appropriate ways to treat the dying: "No one needs to die alone or in pain"; "We will do nothing to postpone or hasten death"; and so on. But there is something about taking the rhetorical high ground (like insisting that "Hospice affirms life," as if others do not) that, while evocative and helpful in speaking to a range of the concerns people have, nonetheless tends to close off other possible approaches. If this criticism is fair, it is reminiscent of the way that invoking God in religious debates eliminates the chance to explore alternatives. This may be what Hospice wants, but it is bound to limit the effectiveness of Hospice in a liberal-democratic and diverse society such as ours.

PROFILE: DAME CICELY SAUNDERS[86]

A tall, almost stately, figure, Dame Cicely Saunders comes striding down the hallway toward me. She is a plain woman, in her seventies; the years are beginning to show. Though her outward manner is friendly, there is a businesslike briskness about her; I worry whether I will be taking up an undue amount of her time. She is, I know, a very busy woman and not a little preoccupied, I have been warned by staff, by the fact that her husband is quite ill.[87] But once she invites me into her office and we sit to talk, it is clear she is prepared to give full attention to meeting me face to face. In the end, she spends a good deal more time with me than she had initially agreed to or I had dared to hope.

The businesslike briskness mentioned above, a palpable firmness of conviction, and confidence in the rightness of her position are the most marked features of Dame Cicely's manner and personality that come across in conversation. She is utterly lacking in pomposity, however, despite the honors that have come her way and what could in a more self-important person be smug satisfaction at what she has achieved and inspired in others. Saunders is prepared to acknowledge that what she started at St. Christopher's has been a "catalyst" for much good elsewhere. Nevertheless, she is concerned that, for example, Sandol Stoddard, in her book on Hospice, is a bit "starry-eyed." Saunders thinks the author loses sight of the fact that "we have feet of clay."

I am struck by the emphasis Saunders places on getting terminology right: "The desperate need is to have proper definitions," she insists as we begin our conversation (as if that alone would solve most problems). "It is very important that you very carefully define 'euthanasia,'" she intones, and "It is better not to use the phrase 'passive euthanasia.'" Since she believes active and passive euthanasia are both wholly unacceptable, she has no interest in arguing about possible distinctions between them. Her confidence in definitions stems from her own absolute clarity on the point. As Saunders sees it, in physician-assisted suicide the patient acts and in euthanasia it is the doctor who acts; she is opposed to both. She gives no indication during our conversation that she is aware of the persistent debates (and disagreements) over definitions of these terms, though of course she must be.

She is equally firm when she explains her own motivation for doing the work to which she has devoted herself for four decades: "I've done it as a Christian vocation," she informs me; "without [Christian faith] I wouldn't have done it." And when I ask for a more precise explanation, she does not hesitate: "God told me to do it."[88] Most of my acquaintances, even those who consider themselves committed Christians, do not talk this way. But given the chance, Dame Cicely does not back down—nor, after meeting her, would one expect her to. This firmness is characteristic of her views on all points having to do with Hospice (and, I suspect, with other things as well).

Neither is Dame Cicely one to worry about her own bluntness. She is convinced, for instance, that the Dutch pay very limited attention to palliative care and that few doctors there know much about it. She believes, too, that there is in Holland considerable failure to follow guidelines or report cases of physician-assisted suicide or euthanasia; she does not cite her sources, but simply announces this as settled fact. Not surprisingly, she was pleased when the House of Lords Select Committee on Medical Ethics in Great Britain concluded that legalizing euthanasia was inappropriate.[89] She is confident that the most persuasive element for the Committee in its deliberations was a visit to the Netherlands, where they saw "how often the line between voluntary and involuntary euthanasia is breached." For Cicely Saunders, there is nothing to debate: Holland is engaged in risky business.[90]

To Saunders's credit, it is clear that her distress on this subject has much to do with her concern for society's most vulnerable populations—the weak, the elderly, the indigent, the incompetent. Her religious conviction that determining the time of death is not a task for human beings sustains her in this. More than once she makes what she considers a self-evident point, that legalizing voluntary euthanasia would soon (automatically, necessarily) lead to *in*voluntary euthanasia. She worries, too, that a "right to die" might become a "duty to die" (thus she shares the concerns of groups like The Arc and Not Dead Yet).[91] In this connection, she considers it a good thing that Derek Humphry's *Final Exit* is not available for sale in the United Kingdom. Humphry, she stresses, "is a very dangerous man." Any book on "how you kill yourself" is bound to put enormous "pressure on the frail."

Similarly, Dame Cicely is at best skeptical about ("hostile toward" might be a better description) England's Voluntary Euthanasia Society (VES), which was founded in 1935. Accusing the VES leadership of fudging the facts to make it look as if there is no middle way, she blames them for propagating the media stories that produce "the usual confusion," leading people to "think the only way to die painlessly is the lethal injection." There is a lot of dialogue, "but I'm not sure how open it is," she says. "Our efforts to talk to [the VES] haven't been very successful; I've been talking to them since 1961."

(Later, when I talk to John Oliver, then general secretary of the VES, I hear the other side of the story. The VES's position is also that the discussions have been unsuccessful and not very open, but it is clear Oliver thinks the fault lies in Dame Cicely's rigid unwillingness to discuss the possible merits of physician-aid-in-dying, on any level. She had said to me, of the VES, "they think we're a lot of hypocrites, that we commit euthanasia under another guise"; when I report this to Oliver, he concurs. But when I tell him that Saunders also said "they hate us, and we don't think much of them," he just sighs and shakes his head.[92] And I recall how, when I told Dame Cicely I was interested in seeing whether a bridge could be built between "right to die" proponents and Hospice advocates, she retorted that such bridges don't need to be built. Thus I find the VES view on who is willing to talk openly with whom the more convincing.

Saunders also tells me why, in her view, Hospice has not been so influential in the United States as in England. Much of it has to do with differences in the way medical care is financed in the two countries. In the United Kingdom, doctors do not earn more for doing additional procedures, and their income is not affected by whether they refer patients to Hospice. Anxiety about possible malpractice suits in the United States is also bound to make doctors treat more aggressively. "Fear of litigation makes doctors do very silly things," Saunders says. But in both England and the United States, palliative care needs more support, more research, more education. Although the approval rating of Hospice is high in the United Kingdom (it is one of the nation's largest charities), full understanding of what Hospice is and does is not always present. Even in England, where the Royal Colleges recognized palliative care as a subspecialty as long ago as 1987, she tells me, medical skills in palliative care among physicians not directly involved in the specialty or with Hospice still vary from indifferent to merely good.

Dame Cicely is rightly proud of what she and others have accomplished so far. I am aware as I listen to her talk that I am in the presence of someone who has had an unusual amount of influence for the good on a great many people. Her indefatigable efforts on behalf of the dying are legendary. Surely she speaks the truth when she says, "we have shown there is another way of enabling people to live until they die." I leave her office and the grounds of St. Christopher's both impressed and moved. Yet I cannot escape the nagging feeling that there is a rigidity both in Saunders herself and (perhaps therefore) in Hospice generally that leaves little room for those who disagree.

HEMLOCK

In sharp contrast to the immediately practical benefits of the Hospice movement's development and growth in England, another movement arose a short time later—this one in the United States—that also has had a profound effect on the way many people think about death and dying. Once again, a single individual played an extraordinary role, as Derek Humphry (also English, though living in the United States then and still today) essentially single-handedly founded the Hemlock Society in 1980.[93]

As I indicated earlier, I am using "Hemlock" to stand for the beliefs of a wide variety of organizations and individuals; thus the Hemlock Society is not our only concern here. Though hemlock was used in the ancient world as a means of committing (presumably rational[94]) suicide, not everyone today sees the most famous example—Socrates's drinking of the poison—in the same way. Cicely Saunders points out that Socrates drank the poison "as an alternative to exile" (though why she thinks this makes the use of "Hemlock" in the Society's name "ironically apt" is not altogether clear[95]). Socrates took the poison because he had been sentenced to die by a legally constituted tribunal. This was, in other words, a case of capital punishment, not the free exercise of any "right to die." Whether he actually wanted to die is open to interpretation; it has been said that Socrates had a "death wish," that he "simply wished to die," and that he "chose death over a renewed chance of life, . . . [a] choice [that] was voluntary, and therefore the equivalent of suicide."[96] Even so, as has also been pointed out, "Socrates' attitude to death and his behavior in the face of it have inspired many"; part of the reason is his insistence in the *Apology* that there are times when "death is better than continued life."[97] In any case, the Hemlock Society itself uses the term "hemlock" in a purely symbolic fashion (as do I). Although "to drink a cup of hemlock" has come to mean (for some) "to commit suicide rationally," dying by actually drinking hemlock is likely to follow an unpredictable course and to be painful, as is carefully pointed out in the Hemlock Society's booklet *Hospice and Hemlock* (1993).[98]

Long before Derek Humphry moved to the United States, interest in a "good death" had begun to emerge. The "good death movement," as it is sometimes called, manifested itself as an interest in euthanasia as well as in alleviating the pain attendant on the dying process. At least since 1938, when the American Euthanasia Society was founded in New York (modeled on the British VES),[99] there has been some degree of favorable interest in euthanasia in this country. Neither mass nor elite support was very visible initially, however, and knowledge that spread during and after World War II of the Nazi programs of *in*voluntary euthanasia certainly sobered many. Despite those horrors, however, "interest in medical treatment issues and proposals for voluntary euthanasia did not fade. The prospect of a slow and painful death caused by terminal illness or serious injury intensified during the 1950s due to the growing ability of medicine to treat illness and prolong life."[100]

Without doubt, the growth of the medico-technological capacity to prolong life has had the biggest influence on people's concerns about their dying. When stories of technologically maintained "life" became part of the daily news diet, concerns that might otherwise have remained private were thrust into the public arena in a way that allowed no retreat from the subject. Heart-rending stories of two young women—Karen Ann Quinlan (beginning in 1975) and Nancy Cruzan (more than a decade later, in 1988)—being kept alive by machines played out on the front pages of the nation's newspapers. The literature on the landmark *Quinlan* and *Cruzan* court cases is vast, and this is not the place to review it.[101] But these two young women and their agonizing deaths probably did as much as anything to raise public consciousness about the importance of the "right to die" question.[102] (Already three years before *Quinlan* began, however, the U.S. Senate Special Committee on Aging had held hearings on the right to die.[103]) In addition, of course, once *Quinlan* and *Cruzan* were settled, new rules of law on some aspects of the issue were established, to the benefit of others in similar straits.[104]

Including more than the Hemlock Society under my rubric of "Hemlock" is important, since several organizations with similar and overlapping agendas exist. In January 2000, Partnership for Caring—based in Washington, D.C.—absorbed Choice in Dying (which had in turn inherited the legacies of the former Concern for Dying and of the Society for the Right to Die).[105] Compassion in Dying, a Washington state organization, played a critical role in one of the two "right to die" cases that went before the Supreme Court in 1997. The executive director at the time was the Unitarian minister Ralph Mero; with his move to Massachusetts, the organization's national office shifted to Portland, Oregon, with Barbara Coombs Lee as the new executive director, where it continues to advocate for the rights of dying patients through legislative and judicial change.[106] In Michigan, the Merian's Friends Committee was formed to help push for legalization of physician-aid-in-dying in that state (the effort was defeated in November 1998), in something of a parallel to the political right to die group in Oregon that pushed for legislative passage of the so-called Death With Dignity Act there. (That move was successful, though the political and legal aftermath of the bill's passage, which I will review in Chapter 4, is still unfolding.) Both who is involved and the specific agenda tend to shift; what matters here are general "Hemlock" principles rather than the detailed tenets of any specific organization.

Even so, the Hemlock Society, though clearly neither unique in its concern with a "right to die" nor the only source of the by-now widespread interest in the subject, has had a special kind of prominence over the years in the United States. In part this may be a result of Derek Humphry's media savvy; more on this will surface in my Profile of him. Today, however, by far the most dramatic and consistent attention-getter in the media on the subject of the right to die, or death with some degree of choice and physician assistance, has been Jack Kevorkian (I will examine this phenomenon in Chapter 4 as well). One effect of the extreme nature of Kevorkian's activities has been to move both the Hemlock Society and the whole right-to-die debate into the mainstream of public debate.

The 1993 mission statement of the incorporated entity, The Hemlock Society U.S.A., specified a belief that "terminally ill people should have the right to self-determination for all end-of-life decisions." It bases its insistence that "dying people must be able to retain their dignity, integrity and self-respect" on a self-professed reverence for life, and encourages, through education and research, "public acceptance of voluntary physician aid-in-dying for the terminally ill."[107]

A short two years later, however, the organization briefly made headlines by proposing a change in its mission statement, saying that "all mentally competent adults"—regardless of whether they were terminally ill—should have the "right to self-determination." This broadening of the mission was enough to make "even ardent supporters . . . nervous," according to one account.[108] Certainly there is a big difference between working to establish "a climate of public opinion that is tolerant of the right of terminally ill people to end their lives in a planned manner" and urging that those who are *not* dying or ill should enjoy the same tolerance.

A few months later a fund-raising appeal to supporters of ERGO! (Euthanasia Research & Guidance Organization, run by Derek Humphry) said that the Hemlock Society had "approved a mission statement which excludes from its policy helping the irreversibly ill. Doubtless Hemlock has its reasons for these changes."[109] By 2001, Humphry was being more explicit about this change on his own Web site. "When Humphry started Hemlock," he writes of himself there, and for its first ten years of existence, the Society's credo embraced assisted dying (preferably medical) for the terminally ill and the hopelessly ill, such as patients with advanced ALS or MS, or extreme old age with severe health problems. But as Hemlock became more involved in state politics in its drive to change the law to secure physician-assisted suicide, it dropped the other illnesses and spoke only for "the advanced terminally ill." While recognizing this as necessary political expediency, Humphry stays firm in his belief that many more persons also deserve assisted dying. This conviction keeps him on the "radical left" of the movement. But he remains convinced that it is never, nor should it in the future be, any part of the right-to-die movement's role to advance assisted dying for the mentally disturbed, including the depressed, nor for the disabled or the handicapped.[110]

Be that as it may, in 1999 the then–president of the San Diego chapter of Hemlock (also a national Hemlock Society Board member) told me that Hemlock's activist efforts are aimed at changing the law so that "terminally ill, competent adults" have choices about when and how to die.[111] That this is a controversial area is made clear in a short piece written by Howard Brody, of the Center for Ethics and Humanities in the Life Sciences at Michigan State University, in response to a letter to the editor of the *NEJM* that appeared in the issue of December 7, 2000. The topic was a report on the clinical condition of sixty-nine of Dr. Jack Kevorkian's patients, on how many of them "had been classified as terminally ill." Brody ends his commentary thus: "The ethical question remains whether the values of respect for patient autonomy and desire to end suffering, said to be the moral values underlying support of physician-assisted suicide, can justify restricting the procedure only to those judged terminally ill. The factual point is a reminder that the term 'terminal' has very limited medical utility and significance."[112] This remains an area of particular sensitivity and difficulty.

In the 1993 Hemlock Society publication I have been quoting, *Hospice and Hemlock,* we see that Hemlock supporters are perhaps less open to other points of view than they generally try to present themselves as being. Appearing there is the rather ambiguous observation that the "Hemlock Society U.S.A. speaks only to those people who have mutual sympathy with its goals. We respect contrary religious and philosophical views."[113] This sounds every bit as rigid, in the first sentence, as right-to-die advocates typically say Hospice people are. Yet there is, in the second sentence, a nod in the direction of tolerance. The result is a kind of laissez-faire attitude that at least some Hemlock folks seem to think is the best that can be hoped for. (On the other hand, some stronger statements, emphasizing the common ground between Hemlock and Hospice, appear in the same piece of literature.)

The differences between Hospice and Hemlock are undeniable. In part this is made apparent by looking at the people who align themselves with each of the groups. Where (as we have seen) a great many Hospice work-ers—employees and volunteers alike—rely heavily on a personal sense of a religiously based duty to care for those suffering through difficult times, Hemlock members and supporters seem much more inner-directed and are likely to be less sectarian. "The Hemlock Society U.S.A. believes the final decision to terminate life is ultimately the individual's. This action, and most of all its timing, is an extremely personal decision." Among the reasons the Hemlock Society does not provide personal counseling to those considering suicide is that "[t]his act is essentially private and familial."[114] The contrast with Hospice's emphasis—even insistence—on teamwork, discussion, inclusion of the family, and ultimately on not leav-ing the patient to die alone could hardly be greater. John A. Pridonoff, the Hemlock Society's executive director at the time *Hospice and Hemlock* was published, listed Hemlock's principles as follows:

Terminally ill people should be able to retain their dignity, integrity and self-respect in their end-of-life experiences. Terminally ill people should be kept as free from pain as possible. Terminally ill people, if they so desire, should be at home with loved ones and have a strong support system. . . . Terminally ill people should have the final right of decision-making authority on matters related to their treatment and the issues which affect their quality of life.[115]

Pridonoff's aim was to show that Hospice and Hemlock are compat-ible, but his attempt to support his claim that the groups merely "divide on the issue *of the degree* to which patients should have authority over their life and death decisions" was undercut by his own description of what each group believes.[116] It is precisely these differences—despite the points of agreement—that make it appropriate to use "Hospice" and "Hemlock" as stand-ins representing the extreme poles in the ongoing discussion about what dying patients can (or should) expect or request in the way of assistance from their physicians.

In contrast to the statement about speaking only to those who share Hemlock's goals, Pridonoff later seems genuinely to be reaching across the divide. He says that "Hemlock believes that it is possible for a termi-nally ill patient to have complete and comprehensive Hospice interven-tion" (it is difficult to imagine a Hospice advocate making a parallel statement in the reverse direction), and he ends his introduction to *Hos-pice and Hemlock* in a conciliatory tone. "We are in the process of dialogue, Hospice and Hemlock. Care and compassion for the patient are of vital importance to both organizations. The Hemlock Society U.S.A. is commit-ted to increased discussion between our two organizations so that ulti-mately the benefit will go to the most important person upon whom we focus our attention and our trust: the patient."[117]

For many people, the whole issue begins with the question of whether we have a *right* to end our own lives: Is there, in other words, a right to commit suicide? What made *Quinlan* and *Cruzan* (and the many subsequent cases of a similar sort that have not received the same degree of publicity) so very difficult is this: Even if there *is* a right to suicide, the two young women who gave their names to the cases were not in a position to exercise that right. And that, of course, is when the issue arises as to whether at least physicians should be allowed to help such patients die—hence "physician-assisted suicide." (Some would argue that if the patient is unable to carry out the action alone, the physician's assistance would become an act of euthanasia.) Consider one brief comment that testifies to the complexity of arguments over the right to commit suicide:

What is extraordinary about the issue of suicide is the self-certainty with which both sides are argued; the one, that suicide is an individual's natural right; the other, not only that it is not a natural right, but is strictly forbidden. Furthermore, the thinkers on both sides appeal to the self-evidence of their positions. Yet, since the right in question is said to be self-evident, further justification of it presumably cannot be given—in much the same way that further justification was said to be superfluous for the fundamental principle of the value of life. Consequently, if conflicting principles are urged as self-evident, it may appear that this dispute cannot be resolved.[118]

The author of that statement, philosopher Margaret Pabst Battin, does not give up, however, just because the dispute "may appear" unresolvable. Rather, she proceeds to explore still other ways in which one might understand a right to suicide. (I will return to the issue of rights in Chapter 4 and to the use of principles in Chapter 5.)

The discussion of Hemlock would be incomplete without a word about the startling commercial success of Derek Humphry's book *Final Exit*, published by the Hemlock Society in 1991.[119] As promised by its subtitle, *The Practicalities of Self-Deliverance and Assisted Suicide for the Dying*, the book was essentially a handbook of instructions for those wishing to take their own lives. Cicely Saunders, as noted above, thought the book was best kept out of the hands of the public. Kristina Snyder, at the time executive director of a local American hospice unit, attributed the "phenomenal sale" of the book "to a fear that what people want and need [freedom from pain and isolation] will not be there for them at the end of their lives." When she then says that "hospice care focuses on pain control," she is of course right.[120] Using that fact to imply that such a focus on pain control suffices, however, is precisely part of what Hemlock supporters challenge. More than one writer has testified to evidence—usually downplayed by Hospice—that there are "failures," that is, "patients for whom even hospice could offer little relief from intense suffering."[121]

Derek Humphry sees the whole issue largely in terms of rights; he maintains that he was simply making available to the public information people had a right to know and use if they deemed it appropriate. He insists the book was "unmistakably written for the terminally ill," and that if people who were not terminally ill used information in the book to kill themselves, neither he nor the book could be held responsible. In response to news about three Massachusetts suicides by persons who were depressed rather than terminally ill, using a method he recommends, he is reported to have said in an interview that "if they had not used my book they would have used a gun, a knife or jumped from a high-rise building."[122] Unquestionably, Humphry has had (and still has) his critics. Casting blame on Humphry—as then–District Attorney of Massachusetts's Middlesex County, Thomas Reilly, did—could be dismissed as so much political posturing. More troubling are the views of widely respected figures in medical ethics circles. George Annas, a Boston University School of Public Health professor, is reported to have said that Humphry "has his own political agenda" and that *Final Exit* could turn out to be a "public health risk" if it encouraged suicides among the healthy. Arthur Caplan, then at the Center for Bioethics at the University of Minnesota (now at a similar center in Pennsylvania) was quoted as having said he thought the book was not "written in a responsible manner."[123] More recently, the book has been criticized for making a complex matter appear to be far more simple than it is.[124]

The furor over the publication and possible influence of *Final Exit* pales by comparison with the media attention garnered by Dr. Jack Kevorkian and his infamous suicide machines. Suffice it for the moment to say that, interestingly enough, Kevorkian's book *Prescription: Medicide—The Goodness of Planned Death* (1991)[125] has never garnered the public attention or had the kind of public appeal that *Final Exit* did. The reasons should become clear in Chapter 4.

Is there a downside to Hemlock? To the extent that "Hemlock" can be identified not only with the Hemlock Society but more particularly with Derek Humphry and *Final Exit,* many would say that the discussion just preceding shows there is a decided downside to Hemlock. If "Hemlock" is understood to stand for a right to take one's own life when one is terminally ill, what are the guidelines for denying exercise of this "right" to those who are not terminally ill? Think, for instance, of the Massachusetts suicides that were arguably "inspired" by *Final Exit.*

A second possible downside to Hemlock is the failure (as some would argue) to clarify what the agenda is. Are we talking about a right to commit suicide—and if so, for whom and under what circumstances? Is a putative right to commit suicide based on another putative right, namely a right to be free of pain? Or is the issue more a matter of autonomy, a right to take control of one's own life (including the time and manner of its end)? An effort to join forces with the most signal success of Hospice— the reduction (if not complete elimination) of pain—has at times obscured the underlying questions of rights. The issue for some is above all how to avoid the pain that most people associate with dying. But many in the Hemlock camp are more fundamentally concerned with issues of self-determination and control. Their questions may *begin* with considering whether suicide is a legitimate way out, but that is merely the marquee item. On the screen inside the theater, other stories are showing, which quickly expose the real issue: Who is in charge? Take away all the pain from a Hemlock advocate, give all the kinds of ancillary support that good hospice care entails, and the Hemlock advocate will still want more: the right to control the story line and its outcome. Thus it can be argued that one weakness (it is that rather than a true "downside") of Hemlock is the confusion that may emerge over what the bottom-line point is. Ironically, stressing the common ground that does exist between Hospice and Hemlock—the desire to reduce or eliminate pain—may increase the difficulties that remain in trying to combine the goals of the two approaches to death. If (as Hospice at times claims) Hemlock supporters misleadingly distort the facts about palliation and thus help convince people that there is no solution to pain except to "check out" of life (which Hospice insists is false), that, too, is a negative feature of Hemlock. But there is a legitimate question as to whether the charges are fair.

Finally, the "cause" Hemlock promotes may have been negatively affected by the prominence in the public mind that Jack Kevorkian has won for himself and his extreme version of Hemlock. Derek Humphry's departure from the Hemlock Society and his formation of his new non-profit corporation ERGO!—for those outside the organization who know about it—may also have looked like a splintering of efforts. At the very least, it adds to the confusion over the extent to which the Hemlock Society itself is interested primarily in education or sees itself in a role of advocacy for changes in the law. Disagreement is hardly news. The World Federation of Right-to-Die Societies has thirty-three member organizations, by no means all alike. Moreover, they have varied agendas, spread as they are literally from A to Z—Australia to Zimbabwe—around the world. Focusing attention here on the Hemlock Society should not make us lose sight of the fact that "Hemlock" as I am using it means both more and less than what this particular organization advocates. For me, "Hemlock" leaves room for insisting that all competent adults (not just the terminally ill) should be free to choose to hasten their deaths. Whatever downside there may be to Hemlock, if claims of being open to dialogue and striving for tolerance are justified on this side of the divide, the negatives may well be outweighed by the positives.

PROFILE: DEREK HUMPHRY[126]

The first time I saw Derek Humphry was at a meeting of the World Federation of Right to Die Societies, in Bath, England in 1994. I recognized him from a distance, having seen his photograph on several occasions, accompanying newspaper articles. Later I wished I had taken advantage of the opportunity to talk with him; I was, after all, at the conference mostly as an observer and precisely in order to meet people. Yet having failed to do so gave me an excuse to visit him at his home, a year later.

The visit turns out to be a memorable experience. Home for Humphry these days is a house and separate barn/study off a road into an isolated area in the hills north and west of Eugene, Oregon. Just getting there is a minor adventure in its own right, and I can't help wondering what made this man who has been so very public with controversial views on a variety of subjects seek out such a relatively remote place to live. In a way it fits, however, with the picture of him I formed nine months earlier in Bath. There I watched him in the bar and lounge area, between and after sessions, as often as not quite on his own. Though I also saw him engaged in conversations with one or another of the small clusters of people on hand, the enduring image I have is of him circling the area as if trying to decide whether to join in or to stay on the outskirts. He has the keenly observant eyes one would expect from an investigative journalist; it was as if he thought he could learn as much by watching as by participating. Not surprisingly, however, given his prominence in the right-to-die movement, he was on the conference program in Bath. (John Oliver of the VES in England identified him in 1994 as "more or less on the radical wing but still the main player in the United States,"[127] and he has long served as editor of the World Right to Die newsletter.) The title of his talk was "The Effectiveness of Literature in Self-Deliverance." The awkward term he acknowledges is a euphemism, but he considers it preferable to "the harsher word 'suicide' on the grounds that a dying person is merely speeding up an end which is inevitably close."[128]

Back to the wooded hillside in Oregon. Shown to a comfortable seat in an area at one end of the large room mostly taken up by the office, I quickly become aware how completely relaxed Humphry is; he has had lots of experience being interviewed. My chief problem comes from knowing that he is also quite accustomed to conducting interviews himself; I am very conscious of being the novice interviewer that I am, watched by the master interviewer that he is.

Over the years, as a journalist, Derek Humphry has been involved in the exploration of more than one controversial subject. Listening to him review his career, from his native England to his present home in Oregon, I quickly sense that he thrives on sticky issues. Indeed, he seems to take pride in his ability to provoke—or, rather (perhaps more fairly), his willingness to pursue the truth, as he sees it, well beyond the point where others would have dropped the subject.

Death is only one such topic, as Humphry's list of publications indicates. This includes such early books as *Because They're Black* (1971), with Gus John, a black activist; *Police Power and Black People* (1972); and *Passports and Politics* (1974). But it seems clear now, even though he still calls himself a journalist and an author, that his third self-designation—euthanasia campaigner—has become central to his life. The list of books he has published on *this* subject continues to grow. The most recent, *Freedom to Die* (first published in 1998 and then updated for 2000), written with Mary Clement, is the best to date. Sober and thorough (if still partisan), it is eminently readable and covers the story well. A heavy reliance on newspaper stories (along with more scholarly sources) gives the book a kind of racy, up-to-date feeling, and shows that the old reporter is still reporting.

Humphry's manner as he talks about his career and what he has done in the past makes it appear that it is in part precisely the sensitive and difficult nature of the subject that appeals to him. He seems to like challenges. The issue of whether human beings should have access to means of ending their own lives (or assistance from others if they need or want it), without moral opprobrium or fear of unpleasant legal consequences, is a topic from which most people have instinctively retreated. Derek Humphry may have been the perfect person to stare the issue down, to face it with unblinking gaze.

Which is exactly what he did—by helping his first wife commit suicide and then writing an account of the experience (with the encouragement of his second wife).[129] He doesn't talk about this, and I don't ask him. I already know the basic outlines of the story. Later, I again have regrets about a missed opportunity, wishing I had—not least because I know (though he does not tell me this either) that his second wife also committed suicide. To be sure, that was after they were divorced, and in the version of the story that appears on his Web homepage, he simply says she committed suicide "during a recurrence of the depressions to which she was prone."

Not everyone sees it the same way, and I keep thinking about that. Trip Gabriel, the author of an article in the *New York Times Magazine,* says quite explicitly that Ann Wickett, Humphry's second wife, "was not, by most accounts, clinically depressed."[130] She had also been deeply involved in the euthanasia campaign (she was one of the co-founders with Humphry of the Hemlock Society). But after the divorce—an "angry and much-publicized" event, according to Gabriel—she no longer worked for the organization. The criticisms she apparently made in a pre-suicide videotape, both of the Hemlock Society and of her ex-husband, need to be put in that context. Still, her accusation that Derek Humphry had become "an agent of death and dying" is unsettling, at the very least.[131] I find it strange to be talking to someone I know helped his first wife die and whose second wife claimed in suicide notes and a videotape that he had put such pressure on her psychologically that she finally committed suicide, too—and to have nothing said about either event. I should have asked.

Later, a newspaper clipping from three years earlier turns up in my files. In it, an experienced reporter who interviewed Humphry after he gave a talk titled "The Debate Over the Right to Die" at the annual meeting of the American Society on Aging (in San Diego, in 1992) admits to also not having asked the obvious questions. I feel better, realizing that my squeamishness did not stem only from inexperience. "My problem," the reporter wrote, "was that I had read too much about the author of *Final Exit* before such a close encounter. Because I knew about the suicide of his second wife, who helped him write a book about the suicide of his first wife, all I really wanted to know was how his third wife was getting along back in Eugene, Ore. It didn't seem polite to ask."[132] Precisely my view.

Part of my problem is that Humphry seems quite prepared to share his views and to educate me on the subject of euthanasia and to remind me of his role in opening up the debate, but he shows no signs of any personal warmth. He seems guarded. Perhaps he has been criticized too often in the press to want to expose himself more than necessary; perhaps he has always been a private person. In well over an hour of conversation, I never feel I am getting close to the real Derek Humphry, though I certainly do learn about the history and current state of affairs in the movement. I can only speculate about what truly motivates him. The best clue, perhaps, lies in the remark he uses as a quotation (he is quoting himself) at the top of his homepage: "The right to choose to die when in advanced terminal or hopeless illness is the ultimate civil liberty."[133]

If this is so, then perhaps the quiet and seemingly laid-back person I am interviewing is indeed at heart a muckraking, investigative journalist. But clearly he has a personal vested interest in this subject in a way that was perhaps not true of some of his earlier journalistic efforts. Despite the direct line from the book about his first wife's death to the founding of the Hemlock Society (in response to requests from readers for help of the sort he had given his wife; the society was initially funded by royalties from the book), Humphry is prepared to give credit to others for the work they have done. The "real pioneer," he insists, was Joseph Fletcher, whose 1954 book *Morals and Medicine* included a chapter called "Euthanasia: Our Right to Die."[134] And today? Asked about Jack Kevorkian, he immediately says he doesn't like the "chemistry," by which he seems to mean the man's personality. "He gives me the creeps," Humphry says—an interesting choice of words, I think to myself, given the number of times I've heard people say they find Humphry creepy.

More seriously, he adds that he thinks we all owe a great deal to Kevorkian. "What he has done," the founder of the Hemlock Society insists, "is to turn this into a blue-collar issue." Where in the past most of the thinking and talking about the right to die was done by an intellectual and professional elite, Kevorkian has gotten the discussion onto the front pages of daily newspapers all over the country. Humphry is fundamentally interested in education on this subject, and in the guise of an educator he has to be pleased that more information than ever is getting out to more of the people who might need it. The right to decide about the time and manner of one's own death should not be a matter only for elites.

Humphry left his position as head of the Hemlock Society not long after *Final Exit* was published. In part this was because he was tired of the administrivia (the organization had grown enormously since its early days) and in part because he wanted to be free to promote the book and respond to the claims on his time that the accompanying media attention created. By no means did his leaving the helm mean he was abandoning ship. Indeed, just months before I pay him my visit, he put out the first issue of a newsletter from his new organization. Aimed very specifically at sharing information, ERGO! is run out of Humphry's office in his woodsy retreat.

He is, of course, tied to the world by phone, fax, and Internet, so this remoteness doesn't matter. Besides, Oregon is a very good place to be for anyone interested in the subject of the right to die. The first ERGO! newsletter blared a bold headline: "Assisted suicide law passes in Oregon: now make it work." The accompanying article, over Humphry's byline, begins with the proud claim: "Truth about dying made a democratic entry into modern society in the English-speaking world . . . when the citizens of Oregon voted YES." Although the victory was narrow, it is one "we are entitled to savor." The "Letters" column has responses from Humphry and a promise that all communications will be answered. He is definitely in the information business. Eager to talk about this new endeavor, he shows no interest in explaining his departure from the Hemlock Society.

I rise to leave. I still have not warmed to this man—nor, I imagine, has he been much taken with me. I'm just one more person asking him to explain one more time how he became a euthanasia campaigner. He has answered much more sensitive and difficult questions than those I have posed. The two hours I have spent with Humphry in no way support Dame Cicely's assertion that "Derek Humphry is a very dangerous man." John Oliver's characterization of him as approachable appears to hit closer to the target. If Humphry seems a bit obsessed by the topic to which he has devoted so much time, he also comes across as gentle, thoughtful, concerned, well informed, and soberly rational. Definitely not scary.

NOTES

1. Merrill Moore, from "Now that She Knows Is Little Consolation," in *The Dance of Death in the Twentieth Century* (Brooklyn, N.Y.: I. E. Rubin, 1957), p. 43.

2. Ken Arnold, Brian Hurwitz, Francis McKee, and Ruth Richardson, *Doctor Death: Medicine at the End of Life* (London: The Wellcome Trust, 1997), p. 24.

3. A recent article included reference to "the age of infectious disease" having been "declared at an end" in the 1970s. Naomi Aoki, "Nation wants vaccines, but drug makers remain wary of the risks," *BG* (14 Nov. 2001): D1.

4. See "Part I: The Tame Death," Philippe Ariès (Helen Weaver, trans.), *The Hour of Our Death* (New York: Oxford University Press, 1991 [Knopf, 1981]), pp. 5–28.

5. Ariès, *The Hour*, pp. 105–07 and generally, is also good on the *artes moriendi*, fifteenth-century (and later) treatises on the art of dying well. See also Arnold et al., *Doctor Death*, p. 25.

6. Philippe Ariès (Patricia M. Ranum, trans.), *Western Attitudes Toward Death from the Middle Ages to the Present* (Baltimore: Johns Hopkins University Press, 1974), pp. 7, 11. See also István Örkény (Michael Henry Heim, trans.), *The Flower Show* [*Rozsakiállitás*], (New York: New Directions, 1982), a literary exploration of a dying man's attempt to star in the show that was his own death, and Ludmila Ulitskaya (Cathy Porter, trans.), *The Funeral Party* (New York: Schocken Books, 1999).

7. Cicely Saunders, "On Dying Well," *The Cambridge Review* (27 Feb. 1984): 50.

8. Paul Binski, *Medieval Death: Ritual and Representation* (Ithaca, N.Y.: Cornell University Press, 1996), p. 33. Death in the United States may not take place in the hospital so often as we think; "death in the hospital is no longer the norm." Edward Ratner, "Ethics and Dying at Home," *Bioethics Examiner* 5, no. 3 (Fall 2001): 1.

9. Erwin H. Ackerknecht, *A Short History of Medicine*, rev. ed. (Baltimore: Johns Hopkins University Press, 1982), pp. 48–49, 92.

10. Ariès, *Western Attitudes*, pp. 85–88.

11. Jean Berger, *A Fortunate Man: The Story of a Country Doctor* (New York: Holt, Rinehart, 1967), p. 62.

12. See Hippocrates (J. Chadwick and W. N. Mann, trans.), "Epidemics" I, ii, in G.E.R. Lloyd, ed., *Hippocratic Writings* (London: Penguin, 1983 [Oxford: Blackwell, 1950]), p. 94. Given the frequency with which this phrase is invoked, it is somewhat striking that neither in the English translation in the Lloyd edition—"Practice two things in your dealings with disease: either help or do not harm the patient"—nor in the Greek original, as emerges in a lengthy analysis of the passage by C. Sandulescu, "*Primum non nocere*: Philological Commentaries on a Medical Aphorism," *Acta Antiqua Hungaricae* 13 (1965): 359–68, is there any word that warrants the appearance of "*primum*" in the Latin version. Rather than it being a matter of doing no harm "above all" or "first," doing no harm is simply one of two things physicians are enjoined to strive for (the other being to benefit or help the patients). I am indebted to Joanne Phillips for bringing this article to my attention.

13. Lloyd, ed., *Hippocratic Writings*, p. 10. See also, generally, pp. 9–66.

14. Lloyd, ed., *Hippocratic Writings*, p. 9.

15. Helen King cites Wesley Smith crediting Galen with "having invented the pervasive image of Hippocrates as the ideal doctor"—which she says Lloyd shows was a result of Galen resorting to "unscrupulous scholarship." Helen King, "In praise of Geoffrey Lloyd," *London Rev. of Books* (8 Oct. 1992): 15.

16. Dickinson W. Richards, "Hippocrates of Ostia," *JAMA* 204, no. 12 (17 June 1968): 1049–56.

17. [Editorial,] "Hippocrates Himself," *JAMA* 204, no. 12 (17 June 1968): 1138.

18. Lloyd, ed., *Hippocratic Writings*, p. 67. A variant translation has it thus: "I will neither give a deadly drug to anybody if asked for it, nor will I make a suggestion to this effect." See Ludwig Edelstein, "The Hippocratic Oath: Text, Translation and Interpretation," *Suppl. to Bull. Hist. Med.* 1 (1943): 3.

19. [Editorial,] "Hippocrates Himself," *JAMA:* 1138.

20. For details, see Emil Dickstein, Jonathan Erlen, and Judith A. Erlen, "Ethical Principles Contained in Currently Professed Medical Oaths," *Acad. Med.* 66, no. 10 (Oct. 1991): 622–24. Contrast the claim of Derek Humphry and Mary Clement, *Freedom to Die: People, Politics, and the Right-to-Die Movement* (New York: St. Martin's Press, 1998), p. 198, that "[f]ew medical schools" require the Hippocratic Oath.

21. "But what these men [Guillaume de Baillou, Hermann Boerhaave, and Thomas Sydenham] admired in Hippocrates was . . . the example he set of the doctor's devotion and concern for his patients, and of his uprightness and discretion in his dealings with them. For this example, especially, Hippocrates continued, and continues, to inspire." Lloyd, ed., *Hippocratic Writings*, p. 59.

22. Sandol Stoddard, *The Hospice Movement: A Better Way of Caring for the Dying* (New York: Vintage, 1992 [1978]), p.14.

23. Anne Munley, *The Hospice Alternative: A New Context for Death and Dying* (New York: Basic Books, 1983), p. 28.

24. See Cathy Siebold, *The Hospice Movement: Easing Death's Pains* (New York: Twayne, 1992). See also Stoddard, *Hospice Movement*, pp. 15–46, for more information on the history of early hospices.

25. See Charles E. Rosenberg, *The Care of Strangers: The Rise of America's Hospital System* (New York: Basic Books, 1987). David J. Rothman, *Strangers at the Bedside: A History of How Law and Bioethics Transformed Medical Decision Making* (New York: Basic Books, 1991), explains how impersonal medical care has become and how remote it is from the early altruistic motivation for hospitals and medical care in general, now best exemplified (some would say) by hospices.

26. Siebold, *Hospice Movement*, p. 19.

27. Cicely Saunders, "Voluntary Euthanasia," *Palliative Med.* 6 (1992): 1.

28. Greg Palmer, *Death: The Trip of a Lifetime* (New York: HarperSan Francisco, 1993), p. 136, identifies Mary Aikenhead as the founder, without comment or explanation. She was one of the Sisters of Charity, and a co-worker of Florence Nightingale, who "founded in Dublin . . . a place of shelter for the incurably ill and called it, in English, a *hospice*." Stoddard, *Hospice Movement*, p. 80.

29. See, e.g., Cicely Saunders, "Foreword," in Inge B. Corless, Barbara B. Germino, and Mary Pittman, eds., *Dying, Death, and Bereavement: Theoretical Perspectives and Other Ways of Knowing* (Boston: Jones and Bartlett, 1994), p. xii; also Robert Kastenbaum, "Dame Cicely Saunders: An Omega Interview," *Omega* 27, no. 4 (1993): 263–69.

30. Florence Wald, "Finding a Way to Give Hospice Care," in Corless, Germino, and Pittman, eds., *Dying, Death, and Bereavement*, pp. 34–37; also Munley, *Hospice Alternative*, and Stoddard, *Hospice Movement*, generally. See further my Profile of Saunders later in this chapter.

31. Kastenbaum, "Interview," *Omega:* 264, 265.

32. Saunders, "Foreword," in Corless, Germino, and Pittman, eds., *Dying, Death, and Bereavement,* p. xii.

33. Kastenbaum, "Interview," *Omega:* 264, 265.

34. Siebold, *Hospice Movement,* pp. 26, 27, 37.

35. Munley, *Hospice Alternative,* p. 79.

36. Quoted by Munley, *Hospice Alternative,* p. 334.

37. See *http://NHPCO.org.* The organization's national headquarters is at 1700 Diagonal Road, Suite 625, Alexandria, Virginia 22314.

38. Vincent Mor, David S. Greer, and Robert Kastenbaum, eds., *The Hospice Experiment* (Baltimore: Johns Hopkins University Press, 1988), p. 9.

39. *Washington et al. v. Glucksberg,* 521 U.S. 702 (1997); *Vacco v. Quill,* 521 U.S. 793 (1997).

40. "Varied Groups Set an Agenda For the Dying," *NYT* (8 Jan. 1997): A13.

41. Ira Byock, *Dying Well: The Prospect for Growth at the End of Life* (New York: Riverhead Books, 1997), p. xiv.

42. Katie Baer, "Dying with Dignity: A Guide to Hospice Care," *Harvard Health Letter* (Apr. 1993): 10.

43. See, e.g., the eight-page pamphlet "Drug Control of Common Symptoms" (1990) compiled by Mary Baines (a St. Christopher's physician), a detailed description of various common problems dying patients experience and how to deal with them. According to the pamphlet, morphine "remains the most useful strong analgesic." There is also a section on "Problems with Morphine" and a chart detailing six possible "Alternatives to Oral Morphine."

44. Munley, *Hospice Alternative,* p. 320.

45. See, e.g., a June 1998 pamphlet put out by the NHO, with an opening paragraph that includes the following statement: "Hospice care is palliative rather than curative . . . so that a person may live the last days of life fully." The front cover of another NHO pamphlet, "Hospice: A special kind of caring," is graced with the line "You matter to the last moment of your life."

46. See, e.g., Valerie Grove, "Lessons in life and death," *The [London] Times* (8 June 1999): 18.

47. Cicely Saunders, personal communication.

48. Laurie Tarkan, "New Efforts Against an Old Foe: Pain," *NYT* (26 Dec. 2000): D3.

49. June Dahl, "How to get effective pain treatment," *Monterey [California] County Herald* (1 Oct. 2001): D1.

50. Joanne Lynn, "Travels in the Valley of the Shadow," in Howard Spiro et al., eds., *Empathy and the Practice of Medicine* (New Haven, Conn.: Yale University Press, 1993), pp. 40, 42.

51. Tony Walter, *The Revival of Death* (London: Routledge, 1994), p. 90.

52. Stoddard, *Hospice Movement,* p. 60.

53. Stoddard, *Hospice Movement,* p. 90.

54. Lynn, "Travels," in Spiro et al., *Empathy,* p. 45.

55. Experience shows Hospice nurses can be so focused on their sense that pain should be dealt with—despite a patient's insistence on being left to face the suffering in her own way—that they practically have to be fought off. Janet Peck, personal communication.

56. Palmer, *Death: The Trip*, p. 147.

57. Siebold, *Hospice Movement*, p. 27.

58. Siebold, *Hospice Movement*, pp. 164–84.

59. Siebold, *Hospice Movement*, pp. 178, 187. Saunders says there are hospice programs in sixty countries. How many she claims as direct outgrowths of the work at St. Christopher's is unclear; Kastenbaum, "Interview," *Omega:* 268.

60. Walter, *Revival*, pp. 87, 88, 89.

61. Lynn, "Travels," in Spiro et al., *Empathy*, pp. 47, 51–52.

62. Beth Virnig, "Hospice Use and the Medicare Program: Use, Options for Change, Unanswered Questions," *Bioethics Examiner* 4, no. 3 (Fall 2000): 1.

63. The organization's address is 4125 Albemarle Street, NW, Suite 210, Washington, D. C. 20016.

64. ABCD, *The Advocate's Guide to Better End-of-Life Care: Physician-Assisted Suicide and Other Important Issues* (Washington, D.C.: ABCD, 1997), p. 2.

65. Lynn, "Travels," in Spiro et al., *Empathy*, p. 53.

66. Margaret Robbins, *Evaluating Palliative Care: Establishing the Evidence Base* (Oxford: Oxford University Press, 1998), pp. 16–18, 92–93, and generally.

67. See Florence S. Wald, "The Emergence of Hospice Care in the United States," in Howard M. Spiro, Mary G. McCrea Curnen, and Lee Palmer Wandel, eds., *Facing Death: Where Culture, Religion, and Medicine Meet* (New Haven, Conn.: Yale University Press, 1996), pp. 81–89; also Stoddard, *Hospice Movement*, pp. 146–80.

68. Mor, Greer, and Kastenbaum, eds., *Hospice Experiment*, pp. 9, 13.

69. "Varied Groups Set an Agenda For the Dying," *NYT* (8 Jan. 1997): A13.

70. Although only some 2,900 hospice professionals and volunteers belong to the National Council of Hospice Professionals, a significant drop from 5,000 members in 1999, the number of hospices has gone up dramatically. In March 1999, there were 2,400 nationwide (according to the NHO Web site at the time), but the data-set for the year 2000 shows an increase to 3,368. I am indebted to Scott Vickers of the NHPCO for providing me with these recent numbers.

71. A husband's account (written shortly after his wife's death) of the couple's experience with Hospice makes vivid both his sense of relief and her reluctance "to accept the idea that the battle was over"—which is what calling in Hospice signaled to both of them. Ross Putnam, personal communication.

72. A Hospice executive director writes that he "applaud[s] the promotion of hospice care in the media. Promoting compassionate palliative care to the general public is essential." John L. Miller, "Hospice care or assisted suicide: A false dichotomy," *Am. Jrnl. of Hospice & Palliative Care* (May/June 1997): 132.

73. Russell K. Portenoy, "Palliative care," *Monterey [Calif.] County Herald* (1 Oct. 2001): D4.

74. Douglas Frantz, "Hospice Boom Is Giving Rise To New Fraud," *NYT* (10 May 1998): 1, 18, shows hospice care as the fastest-growing segment of the Medicare budget.

75. See Anastasia Toufexis, "A Conversation with Kathleen Foley: Pioneer in the Battle to Avert Needless Pain and Suffering," *NYT* (6 Nov. 2001): D5.

76. Siebold, *Hospice Movement*, p. 190.

77. David M. Shribman, "One Nation Under God," *BG Mag.* (10 Jan. 1999): 20.

78. Palmer, *Death: The Trip,* p. 142.

79. Walter, *Revival,* p. 89. See the detailed analysis of this tension, pp. 121–37.

80. Beverly McNamara, Charles Waddell, and Margaret Colvin, "The Institutionalization of the Good Death," *Soc. Sci. & Med.* 39, no. 11 (1994): 1504, 1506. See also David Clark, "The script we all have to read," *Times Higher* (28 Apr. 2000): 27, a review of Clive Seale, *Constructing Death: The Sociology of Dying and Bereavement* (Cambridge: Cambridge University Press, 2000); Clark emphasizes the importance of Seale's examination of "currently available 'scripts' for dying." Jane E. Seymour, "Revisiting medicalisation and 'natural' death, *Soc. Sci. & Med.* 49, no. 5 (Sept. 1999): 693, also comments on the "persuasiveness of the hospice 'way.'"

81. Munley, *Hospice Alternative,* pp. 80, 81.

82. Timothy Quill, personal communication.

83. Arlene Lowney, executive director at Hospice of Cambridge (Massachusetts), made a highly professional presentation about Hospice in my course, "Death and Dying in the 1990s," at Tufts University. What most of the students "heard" was: "Come to Hospice and die *our* way."

84. I am indebted to Judy List for making the arrangements and to the staff and volunteers for their time during two days I spent in formal interviews and informal conversations at Benton Hospice Service in Corvallis, Oregon.

85. An example of the tensions can be found in the juxtaposed articles in Ch. 2 of William Dudley, ed., *Death and Dying: Opposing Viewpoints* (San Diego: Greenhaven Press, 1992). The author of one selection says that Hospice is "the most successful contemporary model for enlightened death care" and "the single most encouraging response to the problems of dying in America today"; the author of the other essay remarks with distress that of "all the 'rules' that can impinge on hospice patients, the most insidious may be the prescriptions about peaceful death." See Patricia Anderson, "Hospices Provide the Best Care for the Terminally Ill" (pp. 67, 73) and Vicki Brower, "Hospices May Not Provide the Best Care for the Terminally Ill" (p. 81), respectively.

86. Based on an interview conducted at St. Christopher's Hospice in Sydenham, London, on December 14, 1994.

87. Saunders's husband died in 1995.

88. When I later read in *Who's Who 1999* that Saunders, along with classical music, lists ethics and theology as her "recreations," I am confirmed in my judgment that she finds life a sober and serious business where God is in charge.

89. The report was announced on 17 February 1994. For a response from the VES, see Colin Brewer, "The House of Lords Select Committee on Medical Ethics reports" and the anonymous "The Report in Detail," *VES* (newsletter of VES), no. 51 (Apr. 1994): 1–2 and 2–3, respectively.

90. Brewer, an English physician and member of VES, pointed out that the Lords Committee, by "omitting the vital adjective 'voluntary' as they have done . . . almost throughout the report . . . perpetuated the main source of moral and philosophical confusion in this debate." Brewer, "House of Lords," *VES:* 1.

91. Dame Cicely's expressions of anxiety that a "right to die" might become a "duty to die" appear frequently. See, e.g., her "On Dying Well," *The Cambridge Review:* 50; "Voluntary Euthanasia," *Palliative Med.:* 3; and her (letter to the editor),

"Enforced death: enforced life," *Jrnl. of Med. Ethics* 18, no. 1 (Mar. 1992): 48. For an assessment of the possibility that there might be a "duty to die," see John Hardwig, "Is There a Duty to Die?" *HCR* 27, no. 2 (Mar.-Apr. 1997): 34–42.

92. John Oliver, personal communication.

93. For some of what led to the formation of this Society, see Marie E. Trepkowski, ed., *Hospice and Hemlock: Retaining Dignity, Integrity and Self-Respect in End-of-Life Decisions* (Eugene, Ore.: The Hemlock Society, 1993); and, more recently, Cecil McIver, *Assisted Dying as a Moral and Ethical Choice: A Physician's View* (Denver, Colo.: The Hemlock Society, 2000), and Faye J. Girsh, *Rights of Patients, Obligations of Physicians* (Denver, Colo.: The Hemlock Society USA, 2000). The organization's address is P.O. Box 101810, Denver, Colorado 80250-1810. The Web address is *www.hemlock.org.*

94. Many psychiatrists argue that there is no such thing as a rational suicide. At a conference on "Physician Assisted Suicide: Clinical and Ethical Perspectives" at McLean Hospital in Belmont, Massachusetts (in 1992), psychiatrist John T. Maltsberger took very much this line. A more accommodating view was expressed years ago by no less-esteemed a psychiatrist than Viktor Frankl: "Even we psychiatrists expect the reactions of a man to an abnormal situation [such as impending death] . . . to be abnormal in proportion to the degree of his normality." Viktor E. Frankl, *Man's Search for Meaning* (New York: Simon & Schuster [Pocket Books], 1984), pp. 38–39.

95. Cicely Saunders, "Voluntary Euthanasia," *Palliative Med.*: 5.

96. I. F. Stone, *The Trial of Socrates* (Boston: Little, Brown, 1988), pp. 189, 192, 195.

97. C.D.C. Reeve, *Socrates in the Apology: An Essay on Plato's Apology of Socrates* (Indianapolis: Hackett, 1989), pp. 180, 182.

98. Trepkowski, ed., *Hospice and Hemlock,* p. 29.

99. Henry R. Glick, *The Right to Die: Policy Innovation & Its Consequences* (New York: Columbia University Press, 1992), p. 54.

100. Glick, *Right to Die,* pp. 57–58; in general, see pp. 53–91, for an overview of the Hemlock Society's antecedents.

101. *In re Quinlan,* 70 N.J. 10, 335 A.2d 647 (1976) and *Cruzan v. Director, Missouri Department of Health,* 497 U.S. 261, 110 S.Ct. 2841 (1990).

102. The courts eventually allowed both women to be taken off life support, but it took Quinlan several more years to die; her parents did not want artificial nutrition and hydration stopped. See, e.g., Ronald Sullivan, "'Right to Die' Rule in Terminal Cases Widened in Jersey," *NYT* (18 Jan. 1985): A1, B2.

103. Glick, *Right to Die,* pp. 67–68, where Table 3.1 ("Major Events in the Right to Die") appears. Glick begins his list with the Vatican declaration on euthanasia (distinguishing "ordinary" and "extraordinary" means for sustaining life) in 1957; curiously, he includes the formation of the Euthanasia Educational Council in 1967 and the transmogrification of the Euthanasia Society into the Society for the Right to Die in 1974, but not the founding of the Hemlock Society in 1980.

104. See, e.g., my account of the dénouement of the Paul Brophy case in Massachusetts, "Where is the Boundary Between Life and Death?" *Thanatos* 12, no. 2 (Summer 1987): 11–12. The whole Brophy saga is reviewed in John H. Kenney, "Ruling will let comatose man die," *BG* (12 Sept. 1986): 1, 87, and accompanying pieces by Ray Richard and Richard A. Knox, 87.

105. Credit for having "invented" living wills in 1967 is given to Choice in Dying by Marjorie B. Zucker and Howard D. Zucker, eds., *Medical Futility and the Evaluation of Life-Sustaining Interventions* (Cambridge: Cambridge University Press, 1977), p. vii. "Partnership For Caring" is located at 1620 Eye Street, NW, Suite 202, Washington, D.C. 20006.

106. Compassion in Dying Federation is located at 6312 SW Capitol Highway, #415, Portland, Oregon 97201; the Web address is *www.compassionindying.org.*

107. Trepkowski, ed., *Hospice and Hemlock,* 27; much of the information that follows in my text comes from this 1993 publication.

108. Carol J. Casteneda, "Group may split over right-to-die," *USA Today* (2 June 1995): 3A.

109. Derek Humphry, "ERGO!" (newsletter), Sept. 1995.

110. See Humphry's homepage on the Web, at *http://www.FinalExit.org/dhumphry.*

111. Sallie Troy, personal communication.

112. Howard Brody, "Assisted Suicide for those Not Terminally Ill," *HCR* 31, no. 1 (Jan.-Feb. 2001): 7.

113. Trepkowski, ed., *Hospice and Hemlock,* 27.

114. Trepkowski, ed., *Hospice and Hemlock,* 27, 30.

115. John A. Pridonoff, "Introduction," in Trepkowski, ed., *Hospice and Hemlock,* p. i.

116. Pridonoff, "Introduction," in Trepkowski, ed., *Hospice and Hemlock,* pp. i–ii.

117. Pridonoff, "Introduction," in Trepkowski, ed., *Hospice and Hemlock,* p. ii.

118. Margaret Pabst Battin, *Ethical Issues in Suicide* (Englewood Cliffs, N.J.: Prentice-Hall, 1982), p. 185. See also Michael Biskup, *Suicide: Opposing Viewpoints* (San Diego, Calif.: Greenhaven, 1992).

119. As noted earlier, by February of 1992, already more than one-half million copies had sold; Tom Coakley, "Author: Book not to blame in 3 suicides," *BG* (1 Feb. 1992): 25. Three years later, another writer reported that Derek Humphry's publisher claimed that sales of *Final Exit* had grown from 520,000 to 645,000. "Every month well over one thousand people still buy his book of recipes for suicide." Lonny Shavelson, *A Chosen Death: The Dying Confront Assisted Suicide* (Berkeley: University of California Press, 1998 [New York: Simon & Schuster, 1995]), pp. 230–31. These figures appeared already in the 1995 edition of Shavelson's book.

120. Kristina Snyder, "Hospice Care," *Jrnl. Geriatric Psychiatry* 26, no. 1 (1993): 56.

121. Shavelson, *Chosen Death,* p. 209.

122. Tom Coakley, "Author: Book not to blame," *BG*: 25.

123. Jack Sullivan, "3 Middlesex County deaths linked to book on suicide," *BG* (31 Jan. 1992): 13, 16.

124. Timothy Quill, personal communication.

125. Jack Kevorkian, *Prescription: Medicide—The Goodness of Planned Death* (Buffalo, N.Y.: Prometheus Books, 1991).

126. Based on an interview conducted at Derek Humphry's home outside Junction City, Oregon, on June 21, 1995.

127. John Oliver, personal communication.

128. See Conference Proceedings, *Whose Death is it Anyway? Medical decisions at the end of life,* Bath, England (World Federation of Right to Die Societies, 10th International Conference, 1994), p. 22, for a précis of Humphry's talk. A few years later Humphry said "self-deliverance" was a euphemism that obscured real issues and that honesty required using the phrase "physician-assisted suicide." Humphry and Clement, *Freedom to Die,* p. 7.

129. See Derek Humphry (with Ann Wickett), *Jean's Way* (New York: Quartet Books, 1978).

130. Trip Gabriel, "A Fight to the Death," *NYT Mag.* (8 Dec. 1991): 47.

131. Gabriel, "A Fight to the Death," *NYT Mag.*: 47.

132. Jean Dietz, "'Final Exit' author Humphry sparks debate on physician-assisted suicide," *BG* (12 Apr. 1992): B26.

133. See *http://www.FinalExit.org/dhumphry.*

134. Joseph Fletcher, *Morals and Medicine* (Boston: Beacon Press, 1954), pp. 172–210.

3

Whose Death Is It, Anyway?

Vex not his ghost. O, let him pass, he hates him
That would upon the rack of this tough world
Stretch him out longer.

—William Shakespeare[1]

In the preceding pages, some shared preoccupations between the Hospice and the Hemlock movements have emerged, despite the differences that typically draw most of the attention. Hospice and Hemlock advocates alike are concerned above all with making the last months, weeks, days, or hours of life as fulfilling as possible. Both also see pain management as a central issue in keeping the final stretch of life from being marked essentially by distress and despair on top of physical or mental deterioration. And no one from Hemlock is likely to argue against the Hospice principles that people should not have to die alone or in pain (assuming they do not want to).

Unsurprisingly, then, at least some Hemlock adherents stress their affinity with Hospice supporters by emphasizing that they, too, see the need for better palliative care. The shared concern is genuine and establishes an important meeting ground. Yet the typical Hospice supporter believes that removal of pain is a critical component of enabling the dying person to live fully to the end and to face the process of dying with greater equanimity than is possible for someone wracked with pain, whereas the Hemlock supporter tends to believe that removal of pain does not speak to the central issue. Most Hemlock supporters, though quite happy to be free of pain in the dying process (or at least to have it managed more adequately), are not content to leave it at that. Within Hemlock, the critical issue is rather that one should have the freedom and autonomy to decide when and how to end one's own life: Whose death is it, anyway? Hospice devotees are less likely to ask that question, because of their conviction that the Hospice approach already allows dying persons to make their own choices, to play the protagonist's role.

The differences in response to "Whose death is it, anyway?" give evidence of the philosophical divide between the two movements. This makes the common ground that does exist all the more important, but it also makes understanding where the boundaries of agreement lie essential. Only then will it be possible to reduce the significance of the remaining gulf. A central task is sorting out the matter of rights: What are they? Who has them? How do they fit into the overall pattern of our choices concerning living and dying?

The answers to those questions are best found through close philosophical analysis. Although philosophy may once have seemed the private domain of academic philosophers, today non-philosophers debate many of the most stubborn questions involving ethical principles in the popular press. Definitions of life and death, attempts to settle when the one ends and the other begins, and the morally appropriate way to approach decisions about the end of life have all become standard fare not only in classrooms, but also on radio talk shows and television, in boardrooms and hospital operating rooms.

These are philosophical issues. The extraordinary growth in the degree of concern that ordinary people have begun to express about rights—individual rights at first, and more recently, international and universal human rights—has, however, put "rights" on the popular media agenda in new ways.[2] The United States has long been viewed as a place where an individual's right to pursue his or her goals is largely unfettered. Nonetheless, it was really in the Civil Rights Movement of the 1960s that social issues of a wide variety coalesced sufficiently to inspire a larger-than-ever segment of the population to contemplate the nature of personal rights.[3]

Meanwhile, concerns about health issues of many sorts increased as the health-care industry grew; this is another arena where the debate over rights began dramatically and with considerable immediacy to impinge on ordinary lives. The gradual awakening to the possibility that patients need not acquiesce in every proposal for medical care made by their (often very authoritarian) physicians, for example, was among the by-products of the women's movement. The publication of *Our Bodies, Ourselves* in 1973 and women demanding to be heard by their doctors sparked the challenges to traditional assumptions of physician authority.[4]

The principle that patients had to be given information adequate to their making informed decisions about their health care was actually first established early in the twentieth century in *Schloendorff v. Society of New York Hospital*[5] and re-affirmed in 1957 when the term "informed consent" was adopted in *Salgo v. Leland Stanford, Jr., University Board of Trustees*.[6] Not until *Canterbury v. Spence* in 1972, however, was the "prudent patient" standard articulated. That decision also resulted in a requirement that "all risks potentially affecting [a patient's medical decisions] must be unmasked" for the patient, since a patient could hardly be expected to act prudently without knowing the risks.[7]

More and more people began to raise questions about personal rights connected with health care: What kind of health care am I entitled to? Do I understand what is being done to and for me? Do I have a right to refuse the care I am being offered? Such thinking merged with newly widespread concerns about an individual's so-called right to die when the tragic Karen Ann Quinlan case entered the New Jersey trial courts in 1975.[8] As David Rothman has pointed out, "*Quinlan* took the issue of termination of treatment not only into law review journals but magazines on supermarket racks." And although "the media tended to frame the story as a case of the 'right to die,' . . . many people understood that the real issue at stake was who ruled at the bedside."[9]

That was not all. In *Cobbs v. Grant* (1972) it was settled that a "person of adult years and in sound mind has the right, in the exercise of control over his own body, to determine whether or not to submit to lawful medical treatment."[10] Refinements and expansions of the idea continued to be made. Deciding a 1986 case in which Elizabeth Bouvia, a quadriplegic patient, sought permission to have a feeding tube removed (she could not do it herself) even though it was clear she would die as a result, the California Superior Court not only quoted from *Cobbs*, but also relied on two more recent cases (from 1983 and 1984[11]) to argue that "a patient has the right to refuse *any* medical treatment, even that which may save or prolong her life."[12] In asserting that the "right to refuse medical treatment is basic and fundamental," the court relied further on a privacy case from the 1960s[13] and quoted Judge Benjamin Cardozo's observation from *Schloendorff* in 1914 that "[e]very human being of adult years and sound mind has a right to determine what shall be done with his own body."[14]

Coupled with the media drama that enveloped *Quinlan*, the cumulative effect of these cases was to establish thoroughly in the minds of the public that patients do, indeed, have rights. For some, at least, the move from "if I don't want to be put on a ventilator or to have artificial nutrition and hydration, I may refuse," to "if I want to end it all and die sooner rather than later, surely I have a right to do so" did not appear large. (*How* one was to bridge this gap, even if it was small, was—and remains—a separate issue.) The field of rights suddenly seemed wide open.

Why do rights matter in all this? Philosopher Judith Jarvis Thomson, to whose analysis of rights I will shortly turn, acknowledges at the outset of her book *The Realm of Rights* (1990) that the "concept of a right is only one among many moral concepts."[15] But she also says that how the concept of a right relates to those other moral concepts is the key to rights being of such singular importance. *Having rights is what gives us moral status in the first place.* In addition, having rights has consequences—for those who hold the rights and for others. Because "morality itself is at heart a set of constraints on behavior,"[16] it is the connection between *having a right* and *how we ought to act* that makes rights so important. That connection is what gives moral significance to having rights.

In the first two sections of this chapter, I will examine the kinds of rights we have and look at the putative right to die itself.[17] In the final two sections, I will explore a quartet of the troubling issues bound to arise, sooner or later, in the Hospice/Hemlock debate: the difference between "killing" and "letting die," the connection between that distinction and the "active" and "passive" euthanasia distinction, the doctrine of double effect, and what is meant by the "integrity of the profession."

First, however, I want to dispose of a seemingly minor linguistic matter that frequently emerges in rights discussions, simply because the word "right" is used in different ways. "Right" is one of many English words that can be either a noun or an adjective; if we are not careful, the fundamental and critical distinction between *having a right* and *doing the right thing* will get blurred or worse. All too often, we fall into the trap of thinking that if we *have a right* to do X, then the *right thing to do* is X—or vice versa. For example, I have a right to dispose of my income as I see fit (as long as I am not interfering with anyone else's rights by what I do). Now say, for instance, that I like to bet on horses. Simply because I *have a right* to do so, it does not follow that using all my excess income to place bets (even assuming for the sake of argument that I have fulfilled my financial obligations all around) is the *right thing to do*. The fact that my gambling may do no obvious or measurable harm does not make it right to gamble in this fashion.

To take another example: If I have a (transferable) museum pass, I *have a right* to loan it to someone, say, to Jezebel or to Jabez. But once I have agreed to loan it to Jezebel for next Saturday, it would not be right to offer it to Jabez for the same Saturday. A promise carries significant moral weight; indeed, by promising the pass to Jezebel I have in fact transferred my right to her. Barring other imaginable factors, it would not be right for me now to give the pass to Jabez. To put it another way: I *ought* now to keep my promise; I no longer have the right I transferred.[18]

The distinction between having a right to do something on the one hand and it being the right thing to do on the other should, perhaps, be obvious. Yet much of the roughness in the territory through which we stumble when we need to decide what is right, what we ought to do, comes as a result of the failure to be vigilant in the use of "right." Determining what we *have the right to do* is only part of the task; it is not at all the same as figuring out what is the *right thing to do*.

KINDS OF RIGHTS

Before we can decide whether we have a right to die (or any other kind of right), we have first to figure out what it means to have a right more generally. That, in turn, requires understanding what kinds of rights there are. The single most thorough and thoughtful exploration of the concept of a moral right is by philosopher Judith Jarvis Thomson. Though she is not primarily interested in health care or in doctor-patient relations, her book-length analysis of rights provides a basis for exploring two questions of major importance for doctors and dying patients alike: If there is a right to die, what kind of a right might it be? What are the implications for the conduct of doctors toward their dying patients? In this chapter I will concentrate on the first of these.

Using as her starting point the classic distinctions Wesley Newcomb Hohfeld made regarding *legal* rights,[19] Thomson applies those distinctions to the realm of *moral* rights.[20] Very briefly put, it turns out there are four different kinds of rights, only one of which has the feature we tend to think of first when we think about having rights, namely that one person's rights are directly connected to someone else's duties.[21] Rights of that sort are correlative with duties; if I have such a right, I have a claim against someone who then (as a result) has a duty. This is what we mean when we say that rights imply duties. Such rights, or claims, are "rights in the strictest sense." These *claim-rights,* according to the Hohfeld-Thomson theory, are the only *strict* rights we have.[22]

We have other kinds of rights, however, which are not correlative with duties. Often superficially confused with strict claim-rights because of the way we bandy the word "rights" about are *privileges.* Life presents us with many situations in which we have a right to do X, or to have some Y, but where—crucially—no one is duty-bound to provide us with X or Y. We may have a right to X or Y without ever getting X or Y; no one has violated our rights if we fail to get X or Y. Additionally, we are under no obligation to anyone either to try or not to try to get X or Y. I have such a privilege-right (but no duty), for instance, to buy a ticket to a dramatic performance. I am under no duty to do so, and no one has a duty to provide me with a ticket unless or until I undertake to buy it. Because my right to buy a ticket is a mere privilege-right, it may turn out that I do not get what I want.

Some rights take the form of *powers,* often connected with ownership, or with position or status. Powers are the kinds of rights that enable the persons who hold them to bring about change in the world. The U.S. Congress has the (political) power-right to declare war, for example. As the holder of that right, Congress is able to change the relationship between this country and another previously non-hostile nation into a nation with which we are at war—whether that nation wishes it so or not.

A power-right may also put the right-holder in a position to alter the rights of others or of his or her own rights. In the case of the museum pass, if I give you the right to use my pass, I have altered both your right with respect to it and my own right as well.

The fourth category of rights is *immunities*. To return to the museum pass: In addition to having a power-right to loan you my pass (assuming, still, that it is transferable), I also (crucially) have an immunity-right against your using it without my permission. Immunities are protections against interference and thus against the exercise of powers by others in the domain where I have the immunity. In other words, if I have an immunity that protects me from you with respect to X, that means you do *not* have a power-right over me with respect to X. You simply lack the power to do X (which is less burdensome for you than if I had a claim-right against you; in that case, you would have an actual *duty not* to do X).

To summarize: We have *claim-rights* that impose corresponding duties on others, *privilege-rights* that give us opportunities but guarantee no results, *power-rights* that enable us to change the world around us, and *immunity-rights* that protect us against the power- and claim-rights of others. This four-part taxonomy of rights does not, however, tell the whole story. We also have *cluster-rights*, where more than one kind of right comes into play simultaneously. Thomson points out that "some, perhaps even most, of what we commonly call rights are cluster-rights."[23] A cluster-right may, incidentally, contain any combination of the four basic kinds of rights.

A prime example, according to Thomson, is what we mean when we say we are "at liberty" to do X. I am at liberty to do X if, but only if (a) I am under no duty *not* to do X—which means I have a *privilege* in this regard, and (b) I have a *claim* against everyone to non-interference—which means that others have a duty not to interfere. Here we have two different kinds of rights in one; hence liberty is a cluster-right. This is but one example. Cluster-rights may in fact contain any combination of privileges, claims, immunities, and powers.

One consequence of the prevalence of cluster-rights is that figuring out what kind of right some alleged right is often turns out to be a far more complicated matter than we might initially have expected. Certainly this is part of why talk about an unexplained "right to die" often leads to confusion.[24] We have already seen, for instance, that neglecting the substantive-adjective distinction in the use of the word "right" can lead to misunderstanding. Several steps may be required before we can figure out what kind of right a particular right is or might be.

THE RIGHT TO DIE

The right to die—and whether we in fact have such a right—is one of the central topics in the debate between Hospice and Hemlock. It is generally those in the Hemlock camp who argue that we have a right to die; the emphasis on this right has, perhaps not surprisingly, become one of the primary targets of criticism for Hospice supporters. Many of them insist the burden of the argument should fall on the proponents of the idea that we should allow people to die when and as they will.

In part this stems from the uneasy conclusion drawn by some that if we acknowledge a *right* to die and allow physicians to help patients die on the ground that they have the right, pressure from physicians could lead to patients believing they have a *duty* to die. Among those who take this line is Cicely Saunders.[25] Yet vagueness concerning what a right is and what it means to have one severely cripples the discussion. This is where the Hohfeld-Thomson analysis of what rights are, how they work, and what it means to have a particular kind of right comes into play. We can use it to help us discover what kind of a right a right to die might be.

Once again, some minor but troubling language problems emerge at the outset. For one thing, it seems odd at best to talk about having a right to some process or event that cannot be prevented or averted. The one great surety of life is that we are going to die; a *right* to do so may seem superfluous.[26] Second, for many people there seems to be a kind of implied parallel to the "right to life." Yet a true parallel would have to be the "right to death" (or possibly a "right to be dead"), and that simply is not the way most people talk.[27] That locution is in any case also subject to the first objection, of course; death (or being dead), like dying, is unavoidable. (The parallel to a "right to life" is moreover far from perfect, since life—any particular life—is by no means a foregone conclusion, whereas every particular death is inevitable.)

Some will no doubt want to dismiss these concerns as mere linguistic quibbles, but part of the challenge we face is that those who proclaim a "right to die" generally express themselves in a way that makes it impossible to be sure what they mean. Presumably it is reasonably clear to all concerned that "a right to die" is a kind of shorthand for something more complicated. For some it may mean "a right to die in a manner and at a time of one's own choosing." For others it could mean "a right to die with the maximum degree of self-control" or "a right to die in a way that permits the greatest possible degree of human dignity to be maintained." Or a right to die may not be a *right* at all—because it means only that the right *way* to die is to be in the company of one's family and free of avoidable pain. These (among many possible) different efforts to expand the ellipsis created by using "right to die" make clear how imprecise the short version is. It is preposterous to assume that we all know exactly what is meant, or that we all mean exactly the same thing, whenever a "right to die" is invoked. The casual use of this cryptic expression is all the more unfortunate, given that the topic is such a difficult one and that what is at stake is so momentous.

Admittedly, however, the phrase does have a certain blunt appeal to it; more than one book author has used it as a title.[28] Despite its imprecision, "right to die" appears to be with us to stay, and since the issue has such a firm place in the continuing debates over end-of-life decision-making, I will also use the expression—endeavoring to add precision as necessary to make sense of the phrase.

From the Hospice point of view, any discussion of a right to die is a relatively easy, if negative, task. Hospice simply asserts there is no right to die (as they perceive others to be using the phrase). The sentiment on this point is so strongly imbedded in the Hospice philosophy that—apparently—no argument needs to be put forward, at least in official literature. A "Fact Sheet" put out by the Hospice Federation of Massachusetts, for example, has the following to say about the right to die: "'Right to Die' legislation was meant to protect the dying. The right to refuse unwanted or burdensome medical treatment . . . does not extend to or embrace the right to die with a physician's assistance through assisted suicide or active euthanasia."[29] This, of course, at best barely approximates an argument; instead, there is an implicit insistence that "right to die" is a misnomer for legislation that allows dying patients to refuse treatment—because of course it cannot mean that a physician can be expected to help the patient die. Still, the patient's right to refuse even life-sustaining treatment if the patient deems it "unwanted or burdensome" is acknowledged. So perhaps, if we press a little, Hospice could be said to agree that *if* there is a right to die (which, presumptively, there is not), then it is nothing more than the now well-established right to refuse treatment. If the patient dies for want of the rejected treatment, well, that has to be allowed (as, by law, of course it does).

Another Hospice Federation of Massachusetts document, a resolution passed by members of the Federation in 1995, is somewhat more forceful. It ends thus: "Be it further resolved that the Hospice Federation of Massachusetts neither endorses nor condones the practice of voluntary euthanasia or assisted suicide in the case of the terminally ill." The prose on the national organization's Web site is understandably more discursive, but also more guarded, in expressing the aims and purposes of the National Hospice and Palliative Care Organization (NHPCO). There we are told that the organization "advocates for the terminally ill and their families. It also develops public and professional educational programs and materials to enhance understanding and availability of hospice and palliative care."[30] Conspicuous by its absence is any mention of physician-aid-in-dying.

From what we have seen so far, it is plausible to hypothesize that if a Hospice argument *were* to be made against a right to die, it would likely (though of course not necessarily) take a statement of religious belief as its point of departure. Life is God-given (sacred) and therefore not man's to dispose of; the sanctity of life is such that life should be lived to the end with no interference; the sanctity of life trumps any right to die.

Let us turn now to what Hemlock supporters might mean when they claim a "right to die." This is both easier—because they do make such claims—and harder, because the disagreement about the scope of such a right is so considerable. I will lay out for examination three of the most common kinds of arguments purporting to demonstrate we have a right to die. Of course, I know both that these are not all (or the only) arguments for the right to die that could be (or indeed have been) made and that I will not be able to treat those arguments fully adequately. Rather, my object is to give shape to some of the current arguments (for the most part only implicit) in favor of a right to die, in order then to have a basis for judging what kind of a right it could be, if it exists.

All three of these arguments invite comment vis à vis their status under the law. The first relies explicitly on a settled legal point; the second is reflected in the law; the third argues for a position that is clearly not (at the present time) accepted in the law. Just so, each of the three can also be reviewed from a moral point of view, as an attempt to establish a moral right to die. The first invites the question whether what is legally settled is, also, morally acceptable; the second explicitly invokes personal autonomy, a commonly accepted principle of morality; the third brings into sharp focus the distinction we reviewed earlier between having a right to do something and that something being the right thing to do. I will focus on the legal principle in the first argument, the moral principle of autonomy in the second, and the principle of non-discrimination in the third.

The first argument, then—the premises of which are acknowledged even by Hospice (though without accepting the conclusion)—is the primarily legal one:

Settled law establishes that I have a right to refuse treatment(s) I do not want.

The treatment(s) I have a right to refuse include even life-saving or life-sustaining treatment(s).

Refusing such treatment(s) could be a means of bringing about my death.

Therefore I have a right to die.

The second argument goes like this:

My body and my life are my own.

I have the right to do as I please with my body and my life so long as I do not harm or interfere with the rights of others.

Given that right, I have a right to take actions that could lead to my death so long as those actions do not harm or interfere with the rights of others.

Actions I take deliberately leading to my death do not harm or interfere with the rights of others.

Therefore I have a right to die.

The third argument—sufficiently extreme that not even all Hemlock supporters accept it—begins like the second. More complicated and more problematic, it comes in two parts:

My body and my life are my own.

I have the right to do as I please with my body and my life so long as I do not harm or interfere with the rights of others.

Given that right, I have a right to take actions that could lead to my death so long as those actions do not harm or interfere with the rights of others.

Actions I take deliberately leading to my death do not harm or interfere with the rights of others.

Therefore I have a right to die.

However, in certain cases the actions I want to take to end my life I am unable to take on my own (for example, terminal illness has rendered me incapable of doing so).

Since I have the right to take those actions and persons not similarly handicapped would be able to take them, and since I may not be discriminated against on a morally irrelevant basis (such as my being incapacitated by terminal illness from, for example, taking pills that would end my life), I have the right to help in exercising my right to die.[31]

Therefore I have a right to (physician) assistance with my death.

I will call these arguments, respectively, the Argument from Law, the Argument from Autonomy, and the Argument for Assistance. Our task now is to see whether using the Hohfeld-Thomson analysis of rights will yield some kind of right to die.

First, the Argument from Law. Though valid, with legally correct premises, the argument is weak. At best it is a roundabout way of arguing in favor of a right to die, as we shall see, because it starts by talking about the right to refuse treatment. However, although (as I said earlier) this is by no means the only possible kind of argument from the law that could be made, it fits what some people seem to mean when they talk about a right to die. We need therefore to examine it on its own merits.

If I had a *power-right* to refuse treatment, then my exercise of that right would somehow affect the status of the doctor (and others) to render such treatment. But since the physician has the authority to treat me *not* (merely) because of some right held as a function of being a doctor, but rather from my having invited the treatment (my having engaged the doctor), then my refusal of treatment is simply my refusal to grant the right (in this instance), not an alteration of the doctor's pre-existing rights.

I do, however, have a *privilege-right* regarding any treatment in the first place. I have no duty to seek (let alone accept) treatment, and also no duty not to seek (or accept) it; thus I have a privilege of refusing treatment at any time I no longer want it. I also have an *immunity-right*, that is, protection against others forcing treatment on me. Those who might wish to treat me may not do so until or unless I grant permission; I am protected by my immunity.

As for the strongest kind of right—a *claim-right*—it appears I have that, too. For my claim to non-treatment (which can include refusing to have some treatment started as well as requiring a treatment that has already been initiated to be stopped) does, indeed, impose a duty on all others. That duty is to not force such treatment (either its initiation or its continuance) on me. Indeed, one rationale for the right to refuse treatment is that each of us has both a right to privacy that allows us to do as we will with our own bodies and a right to freedom from "unwanted touching" (which is what medical treatments and procedures amount to in the law if they are given without the informed consent of the patient).

Thomson makes the point vivid in her discussion of *trespass*, which she defines as "claim-infringing bodily intrusion or invasion." Claims infringed by trespass are fundamental, she says; a person's "moral status is very thin if he lacks claims against bodily intrusion."[32] The U.S. Supreme Court, in deciding the right-to-assisted-suicide cases before it in 1997, along the way dealt explicitly with the right to refuse unwanted medical treatment.[33] The issue, as seen by the Court, was first whether the liberty interest an individual has—protected by the due process clause of the Constitution—includes a right to commit suicide; and, second, whether that right, if it exists, includes a right to assistance in committing suicide. The Court decided in the negative (a topic to which we will return in the next chapter).

Thus, in the Argument from Law, it appears that we do have a right—in fact a *cluster-right*, comprising a privilege, an immunity, and a claim. But these are all rights that have to do with the refusal of treatment, *not* rights that have to do with dying per se. Dying (we assume for the sake of the argument) is something that may come to pass as a consequence of refusal, but dying is not what the right is about. So, on this argument, the right to refuse treatment is strong and firm—but it is not the same as, nor does it entail, a right to die in any further sense. Those who use an argument like this for a right to die are confusing two different rights, only one of which is sustained by the argument.

A stronger position emerges in the Argument from Autonomy. Here, too, however, it is difficult to see how I can have a *power-right* to die. Only if we can imagine that someone, by dying, can (and does) alter the rights of others can we think of the right to die as a power. Perhaps, legally speaking, your relationship to me is such that your right to some portion of an inheritance (from a third party) is altered by my having pre-deceased you. Then, too, your relationship to me might be such that, morally speaking, you acquire as a result of my death some duty to care for my orphaned children; thus your right to dispose of your time and money, for example, could be directly affected by my death. Still, it seems odd in the extreme to think that by exercising my right to die I am exercising a power-right, as if the point of my dying were to alter your rights and as if my dying alone brought about the change in your rights. From the fact that your rights (and duties) might be changed by my death it does not follow that my choosing to die is the exercise of a power-right.

As for an *immunity-right*, there is an important qualifier in the second and third premises: I may do as I please *so long as I do not harm or interfere with the rights of others.* One can imagine legitimate disagreement over whether I have harmed or interfered with anyone, either in anticipation of or as a result of my exercising my right to die. But it is crucial to distinguish between actual bodily harm or physical interference on the one hand and what Thomson calls "belief-mediated distress" on the other.[34] The latter, however unfortunate it may be, is not the harm that we are morally prohibited from causing while exercising our own rights. (We could not be either legally or morally prohibited from ever causing distress or offense, without crippling self-expression, when the distress or offense in question depends on the beliefs someone holds.) Assuming, again for the sake of the argument, that I have not violated this premise, then I do indeed have an immunity against other persons stopping me from taking actions that will lead to my death. This begins to look like the basis for the decriminalization of suicide, an acknowledgment that persons may (legally) take their own lives.

This reasoning is wholly independent of moral arguments supporting a right to commit suicide, which many believe are so strong that they should override the provisions of any law prohibiting suicide. But long tradition in both law and religion opposing suicide inspires vigorous efforts in most circumstances to dissuade persons from taking their own lives. Think of police officers trained to talk would-be suicides off bridges or high buildings and the way we rush to the emergency room anyone who has apparently overdosed on drugs, even though it is legal for them to commit suicide in these and other ways. And we must not forget that committing suicide may still not be the right thing to do even if one *has* the right to do it.

Likewise, a *privilege-right* seems to exist. I have the privilege of taking what actions I wish, even if they will lead to my death (once again assuming I have not violated the no-harm-or-interference-with-others'-rights qualifier), because I have no duty *not to* take such actions—any more than I have a duty *to* take such actions. There are those who will argue that we do not have a privilege, or any other kind of right, to take deliberate actions aimed at causing our own death. They will say, for example, that as a "child of God" one has precisely a duty not to cause one's own death, a duty not to commit suicide. But this is a sectarian moral-religious argument from those who do not accept the premises of the argument under discussion.[35] For those who *do* accept the premises, the privilege exists, but it appears to be a weak privilege-right. All it means is that I have no *duty* not to cause my own death (though there may also be reasons I *ought* not to do so).

We come then to the question of whether, on the Argument from Autonomy, we have a right to die. If the premise that "my body and my life are my own" is correct, it follows that I am an autonomous person. If I take the idea of autonomy seriously, I have a claim-right to act autonomously; there is a correlative duty of non-interference (absent my consent) on all others. Hence it certainly seems there has to be a claim-right to act in ways that might lead to one's death (though we know that those who do not take the idea of autonomy seriously do not accept this). It is autonomy that gives rise to a moral (not just legal) right to commit suicide; it is likewise autonomy that gives rise to the moral (not just legal) right to refuse treatment. The Argument from Autonomy yields both a right to cause one's own death without interference and a right to let the dying process unfold without interference. Thus the Argument from Autonomy yields a *claim-right* to die, because there is a duty on others not to interfere.

Much the same can be said about a *privilege-right* to die and an *immunity-right* to die. Under the Argument from Autonomy, I have privileges of committing suicide and refusing treatment; that is, I have no duty not to act in those ways. Just so, I have an immunity against anyone's interfering if I choose to cause my own death (whether by refusing treatment or by other means). Although a *power-right* to die based on my autonomy makes no sense—there is no one whose rights or status I can alter by exercising this right—it appears that I am in any case left, under the Argument from Autonomy, with a three-part cluster-right, a right to die.

Yet as powerful as this cluster-right to die might first seem to be, it takes the right-holder only so far. This right means no one has any business interfering with what I might do or omit to do with respect to bringing about my own death. But what if I am unable to exercise this right, unable to take the actions I want to take? What if I cannot (for whatever reason) achieve what I want? (Remember that neither having a privilege nor being protected by an immunity guarantees I will get what I have the right to.) *Does this right to die give me a right to assistance?*

The Argument for Assistance is certainly the boldest of the three arguments I have put forward; it is quite possibly the one on which most people implicitly rely when they talk about having a right to die. As frequent news accounts, op-ed articles, and letters to the editor illustrate, this argument has legal (and political) overtones. (A particularly dramatic example came in the autumn of 2001 when U.S. Attorney General John Ashcroft attempted to nullify Oregon's Death With Dignity Act, though his effort was later rejected by a federal judge in Oregon.[36]) Even leaving aside that aspect of the argument, and despite it being a more complicated argument than the other two we have examined, we may have the easiest time disposing of this one. In the first place, if the alleged right to assistance with my death is a mere *privilege-right*, it quite likely will garner me nothing. A privilege grants me (in principle) an opportunity. I have no duty to avail myself of it, and even if I do (or try to), no one has violated my rights by failing to come forward as I desire. A privilege-right to assistance with death does not impose duties on others to provide me with their assistance; I have to find "a willing provider" of the requisite assistance. If I do, however, it seems to follow from my privilege-right that both suicide and assisting with suicide are permissible. Yet as things currently stand in our society, in the United States both moral precepts (for some persons) and legal precepts (the latter in thirty-five states[37]) deny us such a privilege-right.

In any case, willing providers are few and far between. Today it is still true that willing providers also have to be willing law breakers. (This is of course strictly irrelevant if we are considering only the possibility of a *moral* privilege-right.) Even in Oregon, where doctors are currently permitted to write prescriptions for lethal doses of controlled substances knowing their patients intend to take them as a means of committing suicide (more on this in Chapter 4) and where patients therefore have a right to such a prescription, no doctor opposed to the practice has the duty to provide one. The patient's right is not a claim-right. The prescribing physician must be a willing provider; no doctor is under a duty to be one.

Further, even if the legal situation (for instance, in Oregon) were to change in such a way as to make providers subject to a duty to assist someone to die, the patient's *claim-right* would not be a *natural* claim-right. Rather, it would be what Thomson calls a "pure social claim," a claim entirely contingent on the legal provisions of a given society.[38]

If the right to assistance with my death is an *immunity-right*, that may be a greater benefit. An immunity in effect shores up a privilege, stopping third parties from interfering and thus increasing the likelihood that I can avail myself of the privilege. If I do manage to get an offer of help, I have an immunity against others interfering with the help. In other words, if I can find someone to assist with my death (a willing provider) so that my opportunity to exercise my privilege exists, others lack the power to interfere with the help I have arranged.

But do I have a *power-right*? If we can conceive of "assistance with death" as medical treatment, would my right to assistance be such that I could alter any doctor's right to refuse to render what he or she regarded as inappropriate or futile treatment? No. Even when doctors have a duty to treat (which it can be argued they sometimes do, under very special circumstances[39]), they do not have a duty to render every treatment a patient wants or demands. Clearly I am not in a position to alter doctors' rights in this regard, even when the treatment in question is far less controversial than any assistance-with-death "treatment." If I cannot alter a doctor's rights, then I do not have a power-right.[40]

The issue came up indirectly during Jack Kevorkian's first-degree murder trial (in April 1999). Most observers seem to have believed Kevorkian had no right to end Thomas Youk's life. But then these questions emerged: Did Youk have a right to die? Was his supposed right to die one that enabled him to alter Kevorkian's rights? In other words, could Youk exercise his right to die in a way that altered Kevorkian's rights with respect to ending Youk's life? Only if the answer to this latter question is affirmative did Youk have a power-right to die. And in the law the answer is negative. My giving you permission to kill me does not give you the (legal) right to do so.

Finally, what about the possibility that the right to (physician) assistance with death is the strongest of all possible rights, a right in the strict sense, a *claim-right*? This will not work, either. What exactly would the correlative duty be in the case of a right to (physician) assistance with death, and who would have it? If I have a claim-right to assistance, is the correlative duty the duty to do something or is it a duty of non-interference? The latter is no more than what was already available to me by virtue of my having a privilege-right and an immunity-right. Besides, it is a bit odd to talk about a duty to assist when the assistance takes the form of doing nothing. So let's assume the correlative duty would have to be one of taking some action to bring about my death. But who among the theoretically available candidates—health-care workers in general, physicians in particular, family, friends, neighbors, citizens of the world—could plausibly be said to have a duty to bring about my death as a consequence of my claim-right to die? Would it mean having a duty to assist me in my dying once I start to die? And how is that point to be determined? A duty to supply me with the means of causing my own death, given that I want to die and regardless of whether I am already actively dying? A duty to bring about my death by depriving me of food and water? These are quite different possibilities; none is particularly plausible or attractive.

What about the possibility that the correlative duty falls on a "willing provider"? If you are a willing provider, and I have persuaded you to assist with my dying, then perhaps it could be argued that I have this very particular claim-right to die with the very particular assistance of you, my willing provider, on the strength of *your agreement* to do so. Once you have agreed, I *do* of course have a claim against you that you assist, and—barring extraordinary circumstances—you have a duty to assist. Your duty arises out of the fact that you made a promise, however; it is not a duty to assist that is correlative with a right of mine.

Look at it this way: Suppose Fred promised Ted that Fred would help Ted die. Then Fred would have a duty to do so—but it would be a promise-keeping duty, and the issue has suddenly become whether Fred has a *duty to keep his promise* to help Ted die rather than whether he has a *duty to help* Ted die. Even if we want to argue that Fred has a duty to keep his promise, this is still not the same as having a duty to assist in Ted's death because of any right to die that Ted has. Perhaps it would be a very good thing if Fred were to assist Ted. Perhaps it is even the right thing for Fred to do. Even so, it does not follow that Ted has a claim-right to Fred's assistance.

Most of us probably can think of circumstances in which it indeed seems that the *right* thing for a doctor to do is to assist in someone's dying. If a doctor *ought* to assist in those circumstances, this could well be what some people mean by saying (misleadingly) that we have a "right to die." But notice how a right to die of this sort (with assistance) has been severely limited to particular circumstances where it would *be right* for the doctors to assist. It is not a claim-right; it is at most a privilege or an immunity. That brings us full circle, back to the much more restrictive right to commit suicide. Neither a privilege-right nor an immunity-right to assistance gives us a claim-right to assistance with dying, because neither a privilege nor an immunity imposes on anyone the burden of a duty to assist.

Even when "a right to die" means only "a right to die in a manner and at a time of one's own choosing" or "with the maximum degree of control" or "in a way that permits the greatest possible degree of human dignity to be maintained," there is still no claim-right involved (and there is certainly still no power-right). True enough, we have a right to make these choices: We have (for instance) a right to seek control, we have (for instance) a right to do what we can to maintain our dignity. We have privileges and immunities, in other words, and perhaps some few and very particular claims along the way. But no one has a general correlative duty to provide others with the kind of death they seek. Neither are we in a position to alter anyone else's rights in this regard in the process of exercising our own. Consequently, it is unlikely that anyone has violated our rights simply because we do not die in the manner and at the time we prefer, or with the maximum degree of control, or in a way that permits us to maintain the greatest possible human dignity.

If we were deprived of medical remedies and procedures that were promised, or if we were deprived of the kind of care that everyone agrees human decency requires and that is available, or if we needlessly suffered from unremitting pain because someone insisted on following the rule book rather than paying attention to our needs as patients—then we might have complaints, and very legitimate ones at that. But a right to die would not have been violated, even if we have not been treated in the way that would have been *right,* that is, in the way we *ought* to have been treated.

Take an example: If a doctor resuscitates me despite a valid "Do not resuscitate" order, certainly my right to refuse treatment has been violated. It does not follow from that, however, that a right to die of mine has been violated, even if it is the case that I would have died absent the resuscitation and that I ought not to have been resuscitated and thus to have been allowed to die. Nor does it follow that the unfortunate (in my view) position the resuscitation has placed me in (say I am now on a ventilator) gives me any new rights with respect to dying, let alone a claim-right to die that would impose a duty on the doctor to end my life for me. What I do have, still, is a (moral and legal) right to refuse treatment, however, and a (moral, at least) right to commit suicide. Thus I have a right to be taken off the ventilator (and allowed, presumably, to die) if that is what I want.[41]

So how does the scorecard read? If there is a right to die as spelled out in any of the three bare-bones arguments above, it is never a power-right. In each of the three arguments, we found what looked like an immunity and a privilege, and in two of the three arguments a claim as well (thus in each argument we found a cluster-right, though the make-up of the clusters varied). The problem, however, is that in most instances, these rights turned out to be something other than or merely ancillary to the supposed right to die that inspired the arguments in the first place. The exception is the cluster-right we found using the Argument from Autonomy, though even that left us without having gained all of what those who argue for a right to die are generally seeking.

Each of the arguments we examined has weaknesses, though I did not deliberately set up straw arguments to be blown down. Arguments very much like these are exactly the kinds of weapons wielded by many proponents of a putative right to die. My aim here was to expose some of the flaws of such arguments and to show what the limits of a right to die have to be. That there is work still to be done should also be clear.[42] The issue is not merely "What kind of a right is this right I think I have?" but rather a matter of asking "What is the right thing for me to do?" and "What is the right thing for my doctor to do?"

In none of this have I more than touched on the possibility that *even if there is no right to assistance with dying,* it might nonetheless be the right thing for doctors (willing providers) to assist, especially to assist a dying person who literally cannot bring about his or her own death. That such "mercy killings" (carried out today perhaps more frequently by family members or friends than by physicians) are already tolerated by society to some extent we know from the way some such cases have been decided in court.[43] This is a separate issue from that of whether there is a *right* to such assistance.

For now, I believe, this discussion shows that the much-invoked right to die is best supported by the Argument from Autonomy, but that any right to die is still a fairly limited right because the Argument for Assistance is so unpromising. Whether there might be some—perhaps even many—cases in which the *right thing to do* would be to assist a dying patient who seeks to die painlessly, whether this is what doctors *ought to do* under certain conditions, are matters that cannot be deduced from a dying patient's right to die. Thus this discussion must stand as a cautionary tale whose end has not yet been told—and from which, therefore, no conclusive moral for all cases can yet be drawn.[44]

KILLING VS. LETTING DIE

Another matter near the epicenter of the tensions between Hospice and Hemlock that remains a major source of disagreement appears under the rubric of "killing vs. letting die." This pair is sometimes treated as equivalent to "active vs. passive euthanasia," on the ground that "active euthanasia" is "killing" while "passive euthanasia" is merely "letting (someone) die"—with the clear implication that the former is (always?) impermissible while the latter might (under some limited circumstances?) be permissible. These issues are critical because so many people believe there may be occasions when deliberately ending a life (with or without help from someone else) may be the right thing to do, quite independent of whether there is a right to die. Thus we need to look at what people mean when they talk about "killing vs. letting die" or about "active" and "passive" euthanasia.

Both pairs have become slogans, with all the advantage of easy-to-remember phrases and all the disadvantages of short-cut labels for complex problems. In fact, the vast literature on these two connected subjects makes it clear that very little is clear. Earl Winkler already several years ago observed that there was "a voluminous literature in contemporary philosophy concerning the moral relevance of the distinction between killing and letting-die."[45] The volume has increased since Winkler's comment; here I cannot do more than select for scrutiny a few fragments of the relevant material.[46]

What "killing vs. letting die" really means, and whether there is a morally significant difference between those two acts or between "active" and "passive" euthanasia, is enormously important for dying persons and their caregivers; the ramifications for end-of-life decision-making are numerous. Just as we saw in the previous section that Hospice and Hemlock divide sharply over whether there is a right to die, so too, here. We have seen that Cicely Saunders wants no part of distinguishing between active and passive euthanasia because she believes any kind of euthanasia is killing and therefore not permitted. Not all Hospice folk take quite such a rigid position, but they tend to believe at least that *active* euthanasia is killing. As such, they would contend, it is of course impermissible. The nub of the problem for most of those who work in Hospice is the difficulty of knowing exactly what counts as "passive euthanasia." To the extent that it amounts to "letting die," which might in turn be the same as "letting nature take its course"—and which Hospice by and large supports—some will grant that "passive euthanasia" might be permissible.

The extreme Hemlock position might also begin with the insistence that it is unnecessary to distinguish between the terms in either of the pairs, but for a different reason. Hemlock tells us that even if there is a distinction of importance to be drawn between killing and letting die or between active and passive euthanasia, the distinction is not such that one of these kinds of actions is permissible and the other is not; both ought to be allowed. A less-permissive position within Hemlock might on the other hand insist on a distinction, on the ground that although passive euthanasia (letting die) is always permissible, under some circumstances active euthanasia (killing) might not be. So we have a clear division between Hospice and Hemlock. Importantly, however, at least some of those on each side might find themselves on common ground with some on the other side. Virtually everyone agrees, for instance, that only *voluntary* euthanasia is up for discussion. *Involuntary* euthanasia is murder and is of course not permissible. Yet the fear that "voluntary" might become "involuntary" drives much of the debate over legalizing assistance-in-dying.

Superficially, it is difficult to see why there should be any controversy. The gap between the two elements in the pairs looks like exactly the sort of gap that typically separates right from wrong. In ordinary language, "killing" (other persons) will sound to most people like something that is obviously rarely (if ever) morally permissible. (The exceptions are going to be things like killing in self-defense, killing an unjust aggressor to save an innocent third party, or killing in a just war. These cases are themselves controversial, and they have nothing to do with personal decisions over when and how to die.) "Letting die," on the other hand, sounds like something that is probably not only permissible (simply letting nature take its course) but perhaps desirable. It sounds, in fact, like a description of something that people have done from time immemorial without moral fault.

As for the distinction between "active" and "passive" euthanasia, it might initially seem that Cicely Saunders has it right: The controversy, if any, should be over whether euthanasia is permissible at all, not over what "kind" of euthanasia is or is not permissible. It turns out, however, that even when there is semantic agreement on the key terms, disagreement will remain about what the significance of the distinctions is, never mind about what the right thing to do is. Indeed, this is the heart of the matter before us.

For most commentators, the apparent contrast in killing vs. letting die is one of doing something vs. doing nothing: hence the parallel to active vs. passive euthanasia. But still leaving the latter pair aside for the moment, let's ask: Is the difference between acting and not acting as clear-cut as it seems to be and as ordinary use of language might lead us to think? To be sure, as has been pointed out, English speakers "regularly distinguish without difficulty between 'causing harm or death' and 'permitting harm or death to occur.'"[47] Certainly most of us are instinctively more uneasy with the idea of directly causing a death than we are with the idea of failing to try to save a life. But is the moral difference between acts of commission and acts of omission always so clear? Is there any particular reason to think that, in general, doing what we ought not to do is any more (or less) blameworthy than failure to do what we ought to do?[48] The critical point to consider is whether what the philosopher James Rachels calls the "bare difference between killing and letting die" itself makes "any difference to the morality of actions concerning life and death."[49] He argues it does not, because "when we are careful not to smuggle in any further differences which prejudice the issue,"[50] the difference is not one that makes a difference. If in the end the result—a wrongfully dead person—is the same, then, Rachels insists, there has to be something other than the difference between killing and letting die to make one action worse than the other.

If we abstract this, we get the following: Sometimes precisely because we have chosen not to do X, Y gets done (which would not otherwise have been the case). Do we want to insist in such instances that we simply let Y happen? Or is it not also possible to argue that, in effect, our act of omission—our failure to do X—itself turns out to have caused Y to be done? If so, then *not doing* X is the cause of Y. And if *not doing* X and *doing* Y have the same effect, the same result, then there may be situations (barring "further differences which prejudice the issue") in which it makes no difference, morally speaking, whether we fail to do X or we do Y. If *not doing* X (an act of omission) is morally permissible, then so is *doing* Y (an act of commission). Likewise, if not doing X is *not* morally permissible, neither is doing Y.

Filling in the variables above in a way relevant to end-of-life decision-making, we have (potentially) the following: Where X is carrying out a life-saving medical procedure (without which the patient will die), and *Y* is refraining from carrying out that procedure, failing to do *X* is—Rachels would say—morally equivalent to doing *Y*. A more troubling example goes like this: Imagine that *X* is a matter of carrying out a life-*ending* medical procedure, and *Y* is (still) refraining from carrying out a life-*saving* medical procedure (without which the patient's life will end). Are these two equivalent? For many people, the difference still seems to be important.

A source of particular distress for some people has been the need to sort out whether there is a distinction of moral significance between failing to initiate life-support (refraining from carrying out a life-saving medical procedure) on the one hand, and withdrawing life support (failing to continue providing a life-saving medical procedure) on the other. Once again, the fulcrum for many seems to be the hypothetical point where acts of commission and acts of omission meet. In fact, however, this is a side issue. Legally, at least, it has been settled (thanks in part to some of the cases I have already cited) that it is not (necessarily) any less permissible to stop treatment than it is to fail to initiate it in the first place.[51]

Let us look more closely at the kind of situation Rachels had in mind. An example might be this: Throwing a child who cannot swim off the dock into deep water and doing nothing to prevent the child from drowning is surely causing the child's death (killing the child by drowning). In contrast, failing to jump into the water to save a child who has fallen in (or has been thrown in by someone else) is merely failing to save the child (letting the child die by drowning). Most people are intuitively inclined to say the former is worse than the latter. But is it? For the sake of argument, let us assume that we know the child cannot swim, that there is no one else around to effect a rescue, that we can swim and can safely rescue the child without particular risk, and so on. Now what is the difference?

Rachels's example is even more dramatic.[52] The "killing" takes place when Smith deliberately holds his nephew's head under water in the bathtub (hence references to this as the "bathtub example") until he drowns; the "letting die" occurs when Jones plans to do the same but enters the bathroom just in time to see his nephew hit his head and slip under water, thereby saving Jones the trouble of holding the child under.

What is central to both actions, as Rachels set the problem, is that Smith and Jones each acted *with the intention that the nephew die,* because each stood to gain a considerable inheritance with the nephew's death. Thus the motive was the same (and equally reprehensible in the two cases), and the result was the same: The nephew is dead. Rachels argued, and I agree, that however inclined one might instinctively be to be more appalled at Smith for his deliberate act of holding the child's head under water, we must guard against relying on this instinctive revulsion. Surely, Rachels says, Jones is no less morally culpable just because he has what he must consider the good luck to be spared the need actually to force the child's head under water and hold it there himself. Smith and Jones are equally despicable in wanting the boy dead for their own personal gain, and they are equally at fault for directly causing the death on the one hand and allowing the death to take place on the other. This is not a difference that makes a difference.

Rachels is at pains to point out that he does not believe every instance of letting someone die is the moral equivalent of killing.[53] He convincingly argues, however, that we must not simply fall back on an intuitive sense of which is worse without exploring what other differences there might be in a given case. We need to rely on argument and careful reasoning rather than on intuition, though Rachels acknowledges that "no moral view can escape reliance on intuition at some point." The challenge is "always to be suspicious of [our intuitions], and to rely on as few of them as possible, only after examining them critically, and only after pushing the arguments and explanations as far as they will go without them."[54]

Rachels's original paper, "Active and Passive Euthanasia," opens with a quotation from the statement on the subject adopted by the House of Delegates of the American Medical Association (AMA) in 1973, as follows:

The intentional termination of the life of one human being by another—mercy killing—is contrary to that for which the medical profession stands and is contrary to the policy of the American Medical Association. The cessation of the employment of extraordinary means to prolong the life of the body where there is irrefutable evidence that biological death is imminent is the decision of the patient and/or his immediate family. The advice and judgment of the physician should be freely available to the patient and/or his immediate family.[55]

Philosophers Bonnie Steinbock and Thomas D. Sullivan both challenge Rachels's interpretation of the AMA's position on active and passive euthanasia.[56] They have rather different reasons for taking issue with Rachels here, but both stress what they consider his errors. In the process, they leave largely unsettled the matter of the greatest concern to us at this stage of the game, namely, whether there is a morally significant distinction to be drawn between killing and letting die. Sullivan, for example, ends by saying that Rachels (though not he alone) misapprehended the target. The "traditional position," Sullivan insists, "is simply a prohibition of murder." He thus seems to imply that since Rachels is wrong about the AMA position, the rest of what he says can be dismissed.[57] Rachels, in response, points out that Sullivan does not dispute his argument; rather, he simply "dismisses it as irrelevant."[58]

More helpful is a rich collection of essays on assisted suicide and euthanasia edited by Tom L. Beauchamp.[59] In his introductory essay, Beauchamp takes up the subject of what we mean—in ordinary language—by "killing." Too few others engaged in this debate have bothered to raise the issue, and even Beauchamp still does not deal very effectively with the extent to which "killing" is an inherently loaded term. This feature of the word as most of us know and use it is, I believe, what underlies the common intuition that "killing" surely must be morally more offensive than "letting die." Again I agree with Rachels: We must be careful about relying solely on our intuitions.

Indication of how difficult arguments over killing and letting die are—and why we need to exercise caution before deciding where we stand—emerges from a variety of writers. Although David Barnard acknowledges the strength of arguments like Rachels's, showing that the difference between killing and letting die is not so great as we intuitively tend to assume, he proceeds simply to assert that the distinction is nevertheless "useful and valid both clinically and socially."[60] Another among those who want to insist that the distinction between killing and letting die is "clinically relevant and morally significant" is philosopher Baruch Brody. But he, like Barnard, makes assertions without adequately supporting them. The argument "that active euthanasia is justified because there really is no difference between killing and letting die," he says, "is flawed because it denies the moral significance of a distinction whose moral significance has been established." He goes on: "I believe that we should grant . . . the distinction."[61] This rather begs the question, since Rachels—among others—has cogently argued that the moral significance of the distinction is *not* established; further, in the paper that follows, Judith Thomson dissects Brody's argument, demonstrating convincingly how he has failed to establish what he claims to have.[62]

Certainly Alan J. Weisbard and Mark Siegler are correct when they say that the "line between 'allowing to die' and 'actively killing' can be elusive." They also admit to being "skeptical that any logical or psychological distinction between 'allowing to die' by starvation and actively killing, as by lethal injection, will prove viable."[63] They conclude that withdrawing nutrition is equivalent to active euthanasia and must be prohibited; others might conclude that since withdrawing nutrition is (in some circumstances—certainly at the patient's request) morally acceptable, then (in those same circumstances) if this counts as active euthanasia, it follows that active euthanasia is morally acceptable. But notice: "If this counts as active euthanasia." To a considerable degree everything depends on which definition is accepted. Philosopher Dan Brock is among those who seem to conclude that (this kind of) active euthanasia is acceptable, when he says he believes "that on common understandings of the kill/allow to die distinction, the difference is not in itself morally important, and that stopping life-sustaining treatment is often killing, though justified killing."[64]

We have come some distance from the implied question at the opening of this section, namely, whether the killing/letting-die difference is the same as the active/passive euthanasia distinction. In fact, however, since (as I believe) in most people's minds the distinctions are the same, and that thus to talk about one is to talk about both, what I have tried to show is that neither distinction is in the end morally significant. At least it is not if two conditions hold: The outcome is the same (death), and the outcome is what was intended. Just what we *intend,* and just how much difference that makes in assessing the morality of an act—as the following discussion will illustrate—is another issue over which many earnest and serious-minded commentators divide. We will soon see that, despite the best efforts to find common ground, this divide also separates Hospice and Hemlock.

All of this matters because the linchpin in most arguments that favor marking the distinction between killing and letting die as morally significant is the issue of intent. How much difference one's intentions make also proves, in turn, to be absolutely central to the disagreement between those Hemlock supporters who think that so-called active euthanasia may, in some instances, be permissible, and those Hospice advocates who insist that it never is. Intent, furthermore, is the key in what is known as the "doctrine of double effect" (DDE).

This doctrine comes out of the Catholic moral-theological tradition.[65] Although in 1978 it was still possible to claim that this principle appeared "to be the exclusive property of Catholic moral theology,"[66] more recently the DDE "has figured prominently in the discussion of both ethical theory and applied ethics by a broad range of contemporary philosophers."[67] Its primary use has been to support the Catholic position on abortion, but more generally it "serves the purpose of morally assessing certain actions fairly complicated in their structure,"[68] and is therefore "supposed by [Catholics (and others)] to apply elsewhere."[69] The possible application "elsewhere" is what makes the doctrine important to us here.

The idea is roughly this: Many actions produce more than one effect; some of these effects are what we directly intend to have happen, while other effects may be foreseen but unintended. In fact, they may not be desired or intended effects at all—but they may be unavoidable if the effects we directly do intend are to be produced. Philosopher Philippa Foot explains it as follows:

The words "double effect" refer to the two effects that an action may produce: the one aimed at, and the one foreseen but in no way desired. By "the doctrine of double effect" [is meant] the thesis that it is sometimes permissible to bring about by oblique intention what one may not directly intend. Thus the distinction is held to be relevant to moral decision in certain difficult cases.[70]

Leaving aside the intricacies of the particular debate over abortion, let's see how the DDE might apply to the views of Hospice and Hemlock, where the life one might be ending is not that of a helpless fetus but that of a competent adult. The question typically takes the following form: Is it morally permissible to give a lethal dose of some painkiller to a dying patient in excruciating pain? Some would simply say "yes," straightaway. Others would respond with a more complex line of reasoning. If ending the patient's life is what is directly intended, it is not permissible. If what is intended is simply to reduce or eliminate the excruciating pain, then as much of the (potentially) lethal painkiller may be given as is required to reduce or eliminate the pain. In other words: If the primary goal (the directly intended effect) is for the patient to be out of pain, then giving the medication is clearly permissible. If a secondary (unintended) effect is that the patient will die (because the pain medication suppresses respiration so drastically that the patient stops breathing), that is also permissible—thanks to the DDE—because *although the death was foreseen as certain, it was not directly intended.*

How to evaluate this kind of reasoning, often heard from Hospice people, is a vital issue for anyone thinking about Hospice and Hemlock. A classic example emerged in a newspaper article reporting a survey conducted by the American Society of Internal Medicine, on whether doctors had assisted a patient's death. Loring Conant, at the time medical director of the Hospice in Cambridge, Massachusetts, is quoted as having made the following comment: "I have taken a direct action toward people clearly at the end—by giving more morphine to make them comfortable or withholding an antibiotic. . . . I distinguish that from euthanasia. I'm giving the medication to relieve suffering, not to cause death, with the understanding that it might hasten death."[71]

Does this emphasis on intent—on the reason for giving the medication—make perfectly good sense as a way to justify all and only what one wants to concede is permissible? Or does this kind of reasoning belong in the category of self-serving double-talk? (Is it, in Philippa Foot's words, "a piece of complete sophistry"?[72]) Certainly some physicians stand unequivocally at the other extreme from Conant. "I do not see," wrote British doctor Tim Helme, how "a doctor can admit that he foresaw that his action would in fact 'cause death,' but then claim that he had no intention to kill because he desired something else."[73]

The problem for those who do not subscribe to the DDE, incidentally, is not that they consider "intent" unimportant. On the contrary. But where supporters seem to think that "intent" can carry the entire moral weight of the decision being made, those who are more skeptical of the DDE do not. They find it impossible to ignore the parallel outcomes of cases like those in Rachels's bathtub example. Of course intent matters, but foreseen consequences of something not intended cannot be ignored; we are responsible for both the primary and the secondary effects of our actions.[74]

At this point, the connections between "active" and "passive" euthanasia on the one hand, and "killing" and "letting die" on the other, become critical. We need also to see whether (and how) these rubrics apply both to *what is foreseen and intended* and to *what is foreseen but unintended*. The typical Hospice supporter—the Hospice philosophy itself, it might be said—certainly permits letting a patient die ("letting nature take its course"), as we have seen. Indeed, key to the Hospice approach to care of the dying is the idea that one should not interfere with the process. It follows, therefore, that "letting nature take its course" or "letting [someone] die" is permitted.

Nothing, Hospice philosophy tells us, should be done either to hasten (or to delay) death. Thus anything that can be construed as taking active steps to end a person's life will not be permissible. Whether these "active" steps are labeled "killing," "active euthanasia," or something else, and whether these are equivalent terms, are not the operative questions. Whatever these actions are called, they are not permitted. For anyone who hears in the word "euthanasia" overtones of "deliberate killing" (despite the fact that the word's etymology tells us otherwise; "euthanasia" is simply "good death"), nothing called "euthanasia" is going to be permissible. The labels "active" and "passive" have no bearing. So although to some people "passive euthanasia" might seem to be equivalent to "letting [someone] die," most Hospice supporters will go out of their way to avoid that language.

We have seen, however, that relieving pain is also central to the Hospice approach. And it is here that the DDE comes into the picture. For if one is going to do whatever it takes to eliminate pain, it is virtually certain that, in at least some cases, what it takes to eliminate pain is going to hasten the arrival of the moment of death. What makes this nonetheless permissible for Hospice is the doctrine of double effect. As long as bringing death about—or hastening its arrival—is not what is directly intended, the fact that one foresees this result of one's action does not mean that one would be wrong to take the action that produces the lethal result. This means that you may not give a dose of a painkilling medicine *intending* that the patient should die. You may, however, give that same dose as long as what you intend is for the patient's pain to be relieved *even if you foresee that there will be a second—a "double"—effect,* including one that you do not intend, namely the (hastened) death of the person whose pain has been relieved.

How critical the role of intention is thus becomes clear. Among the concerns we need to have are these: How consistently reliable is one's sense of one's own intentions—never mind, of someone else's? Do we want to argue that basic rules of moral conduct prohibit some actions even if our intentions in breaking them are good and the result of doing so—the end achieved—is also good?

The larger question is this: Is it ever morally permissible knowingly to do something evil in order to bring about some good? That there should be an entire book titled *Doing Evil to Achieve Good* from a Christian theological point of view should cause no surprise.[75] Other books have dealt with specific "evils." For instance, though most of us would instinctively say lying is not morally permissible, most of us would also very quickly want to append qualifications. Sissela Bok, in her careful exploration of lying, shows why we are right to insist on exceptions.[76] Absolute prohibitions of "evil" when "good" might result, like most absolutist positions, turn out to be problematic.

Nonetheless, whether it is permissible to do evil in order to do good is a question that does need to be answered—by each individual who thinks that deliberately ending a human life is "evil" but nonetheless wants to consider the possibility that a "good" would be achieved if that life were ended rather than simply allowed to drift to its "natural" conclusion.[77] To argue solely about "killing" and "letting die" in such instances obscures the myriad details that make each case unique. As has been pointed out by others, there are also risks in assuming that "natural" is necessarily a positive term. "[T]he limitations of 'natural' and 'unnatural' as moral predicates are severe," philosopher Richard W. Momeyer tells us, "and their use far more frequently obscures than illuminates matters.... And where evaluations of modes of dying or the status of death itself are at issue, there is double reason to avoid the use of 'natural' and 'unnatural' altogether."[78]

A classic example of directly doing-evil-to-accomplish-good appears in Plato's *Crito*. A possible reading of that dialogue is precisely the consideration of whether it is ever right to do something evil or wrong in order to fight evil; at issue is the very life of Socrates. His conclusion (to the distress of his friends) is that failing to obey the law—even a wrong-headed or misapplied law—is itself not morally permissible, and so, Socrates argues, he may not break it. This he says is true even if a "good"—the preservation of his life—would come of doing that "evil."[79]

The contrast with Hemlock philosophy is clear. Although "letting die" or "passive euthanasia" is permissible, just as it is in Hospice thinking, the typical Hemlock supporter argues that "letting nature take its course" is often just the problem. The "course of nature" is always independent of and often inconsistent with what would result from the free exercise of one's rights; the course of nature may also create or perpetuate conditions one wishes to avoid. Hence, for Hemlock adherents, actively taking steps to end a life that has become unbearable is also permissible (assuming the individual in question is both terminally ill and competent to make rational decisions). So here is a major difference. Many Hospice people are uncomfortable with the term as well as the concept of "euthanasia" (even when it is "passive"). Supporters of the Hemlock approach, on the other hand, tend to accept "euthanasia" (relying on its strict etymological meaning) as a straightforward—even if not completely unambiguous—term with which they are comfortable. What they try to avoid is use of the word "killing."

This is not to say that Hemlock advocates do not share Hospice concerns about intentions. Hemlock, too, assumes that individuals will act from morally permissible intentions; it is just that what counts as morally permissible is different for Hemlock and Hospice supporters. Note, too, that Hemlock does not advocate "killing"—contrary to what Hospice extremists sometimes seem to believe or want others to believe about Hemlock. The issue for Hemlock supporters is not "killing" versus "letting die," it is not "active" versus "passive" euthanasia (the distinctions are unimportant for most Hemlock supporters) but rather the central matter of rights, the main features of which we explored earlier. Regardless of what it is called—"killing," "active euthanasia," or something else—no Hemlock supporter would argue that the deliberate taking of a life is right in every instance. Most would not even argue that it is right in every instance where the individual wants (or claims to want) his or her life ended. The Hemlock argument is rather that each individual *has a right* to bring an end to his or her life. This is a very different matter.

What should be clear after this discussion is that we are left with several points of contrast. Hospice (in its official literature) argues that it is never right to cause or hasten the death of a person (oneself or others) and that no one has the right to do so. Hospice acknowledges, however, that there are circumstances under which the secondary effect of some action—an action whose primary effect was both permissible and the right thing to do—might be a hastened death. Hemlock, in contrast, argues that whether it is right to cause or hasten the death of a person is less important than the fact that persons have both the right to decide this matter for themselves and the right to act on their decisions. For Hospice supporters, as we saw earlier, intentionally ending a life simply is *not* the right thing to do (though the doctrine of double effect enables one to deal with the awkward cases). For Hemlock supporters, the central truth is that one does have a right to end one's life—which means the question of whether intentionally ending one's life is the right thing to do must always be considered.

Hard on the heels of the assertion that each of us has the right to decide about our own lives comes another question, namely, whether someone else should be allowed to assist in the life-ending action. This is certainly the more difficult—and, socially speaking, more troubling—case. Perhaps not surprisingly, Hemlock supporters are apt to divide over this issue. Some insist that as long as it is clear that we have the right to take our own lives, all is well. Others plead that societal strictures should not be set in such a way as to force the inept (never mind the physically incapable) to try, and quite likely fail, to end their own lives, when competent medical help is theoretically available. (Whether physicians really know what they are doing when it comes to deliberately ending a life, without causing undue suffering, is another important subject, but not one I will take up here.[80])

This distinction between "it is never right to hasten death" and "each person has a right to hasten the end of his or her own life" is perhaps as blunt a way as possible to put the key difference between adherents of Hospice and supporters of Hemlock. Along the way, however, we have repeatedly seen how important vocabulary can be. No one likes the sound of "killing"; few are truly comfortable with "euthanasia." We also have plenty of evidence that people understand rather different things by these terms. Virtually all writers on euthanasia and related topics spend some time defining what they mean by "euthanasia" in particular.

Efforts to lighten the burden these words carry are rarely very successful. Even saying something so apparently straightforward and uncontroversial as that "letting die" is equivalent to "not interfering in the dying process" turns out hardly to solve the problem. Does this mean that the biblical travelers who preceded the Good Samaritan and left the stranger in the ditch were "letting [him] die" in the same way that the physician who refrains from futile surgery is?[81] What about the physician who acquiesces when asked (by a dying patient) to remove all artificial nutrition and hydration? Are these all the same kind of "letting die"? Surely not.

The situation is similar when we use the word "killing," which for most of us carries with it images of mayhem and murder. We presumably mean something rather different when an innocent person is caught and shot in the crossfire of gang warfare on the street, and when a physician, at the earnest request of a patient, thoughtfully injects that patient with a lethal dose of some drug. Even that picture is blurred, however, as Jack Kevorkian's last case made evident.[82] What remains is the realization of how extremely careful our choice of words must be when we talk about what is morally permissible behavior. Even well-chosen words and phrases can turn and twist until they have more to do with propaganda than principle.

THE INTEGRITY OF THE PROFESSION

Those who accept the right of persons to end their own lives may still balk at the idea that physicians should be allowed to assist in any shape, form, or manner. One of the arguments often used against legalizing physician-aid-in-dying is that to do so would be to allow physicians to do something that works against the "integrity of the profession." For an individual to take his or her own life is one thing, it is granted, but it is quite another for a physician—trained to save lives—to participate in deliberately ending a life prematurely. Ignoring for the present the fact that the phrase "integrity of the profession" is itself notably vague and to that extent of uncertain content, let's look briefly at two points that surface repeatedly and prominently.

The first concern for many is the apparent self-evidence of the proposition that doctors mustn't kill. The whole point of the profession of medicine, after all—or so it is argued—is to heal, to make well, to preserve life. Joseph Fletcher quotes (sympathetically, though without endorsing) from a Catholic protest against legalizing euthanasia (and presumably any kind of "killing" by doctors: It "would be a confession of despair in the medical profession; it would be a denial of hope for further progress against presently incurable maladies. It would destroy all confidence in physicians, and introduce a reign of terror."[83] But as Fletcher later says, though we may agree that the physician's ethics forbid the taking of life, still "there are cases when the doctor's duty to prolong and protect life is in conflict with his duty to relieve suffering. As a matter of fact, this dilemma is actually inescapable and inherent in the medical care of many terminal illnesses anyway, at the technical as well as the moral level."[84]

Nothing in the half century since Fletcher wrote those words has removed the "inescapable and inherent" dilemma he identified, even if its shape and the frequency of its appearance have changed.[85] Moreover, the questions most asked today about the effect on the "integrity of the [medical] profession" of legally allowing doctors to end their patients' lives under particular circumstances are by their nature unanswerable unless or until we legalize physician-aid-in-dying (or euthanasia). Ronald Dworkin lists some half-dozen of these troubling empirical questions, but points out that—despite the importance of those questions—we need to think about "an even more fundamental matter: which decision is the *right* one to make, no matter who makes it?" For Dworkin as for me, the "paramount question" is how we should think about when and how to die.[86]

Once again, the challenge of choosing the right words arises. Without doubt, "kill" is a potent term; it is easy to agree that doctors should not be permitted to engage in "killing" patients. But causing a patient's life to end could just as easily be seen as something other than "killing." Ending a patient's life could be called "assisting" an individual who is suffering, or "supporting" a patient through difficult times, or being "a midwife through the dying process." With such language, it becomes much more difficult to understand why doctors should not be permitted (under carefully controlled conditions) to end the lives of their competent patients who have requested their help in this most profound of moments.

A second source of anxiety for those who concern themselves with the "integrity of the [medical] profession" is what is often called the "slippery slope" argument, which says that doctors may slide, bit by bit, from legitimate practices to those of debatable legitimacy to wholly unacceptable ones.[87] At the outset it should be noted that the concern is frequently expressed in imprecise questions such as "What about the slippery slope?" rather than in the form of an analyzable argument. Absent a serious argument, "slippery slope" is a truncheon waved about to frighten the undecided into opposition; used as such, it is a prime example of the propaganda in lieu of principle to which I referred above.

Almost worse is what happens when those who rely on the "slippery slope" to make their negative point about the dangers to the integrity of the profession they believe is represented by physician-assisted suicide *do* take the trouble to spell out an argument. The result is too often primitive and crude. The move tends to be extremely rapid, from hypotheticals like "if we allow doctors to kill patients in a few selected instances" to assertions of certitude like "the profession will end up behaving like the Nazi doctors with their concerted program of involuntary euthanasia." Even Dworkin, in the interest of brevity, allows himself to be satisfied with presenting a very condensed version of the argument, because the details of the argument are not what concern him at that particular point. He does neither himself nor the argument much of a favor when he says that even when the kinds of cases in which euthanasia is legalized are carefully limited, there is an increased likelihood that "more doubtful" cases will subsequently be legalized, with the result that "the process may end in Nazi eugenics."[88]

The gigantic leap from one hypothetical condition to a grossly exaggerated conclusion—rarely expressed as cautiously as Dworkin took the trouble to do (he at least used "may")—distorts the issue. Dworkin also points out that the argument against legalizing euthanasia fails to consider that forcing people who want to die to stay alive may be harmful to them. Likewise, he says, the "slippery slope" argument ignores the fact that legalizing euthanasia is an attempt to establish a defensible position and reduce the risk of less-defensible positions being established later. Doing that, he insists, "is better than abandoning those people altogether. There are dangers both in legalizing and refusing to legalize; the rival dangers must be balanced, and neither should be ignored."[89]

There is a two-fold problem with every form of the slippery-slope argument. In the first place, very little empirical evidence is available of the type that would help show whether the conclusion being drawn is certain or even likely. Second, what evidence there is tends not to be taken into account; certainly those who oppose legalization do not mention it.[90] Why? Probably because most of the relevant experience we have in this country comes from the tightly knit community of those suffering from AIDS who have committed themselves to helping others with AIDS die— not least in the hope that someone will do the same for them when the time comes. One doctor who has become familiar with the gay community in San Francisco has remarked how impressed he was "by how closely everyone followed a set of unwritten but well-understood rules—with no law in place to assure that they do so." Acknowledging that there are legitimate fears about how (some) physicians would react to the legalization of physician-assisted suicide, this doctor continues as follows: "[I]f physicians, given the legal right to assist in hastening death, will be as careful as the gay men of the Castro seem to have been, the safeguards of close regulation and oversight should prevent almost all abuses."[91] This of course also does not constitute an argument, but certainly there is food for thought even in a very small sample of cases that relies on anecdotal data. The questions that need to be raised when people wave the slippery-slope banner are empirical ones, and they cannot be fully answered until physician-aid-in-dying has been legalized.

To circumvent this Catch-22, some have turned to the Netherlands, where just such assistance from physicians was long tolerated and has now been legalized. Holland is not really an appropriate model for us, however, for reasons I will explain in the next chapter. Those who argue as if they know what the practical effects would be of legalizing physician-aid-in-dying here are being disingenuous. Without a true experiment and the gathering of empirical data, we do not—and cannot—know what the result would be, either for individual patients or for the medical profession as a whole, if doctors were legally permitted to help patients end their lives.

That does not mean we should throw up our hands in despair or stop being concerned about possible risks, the "legitimate fears" mentioned earlier. Rather, it means we should hesitate before jumping to conclusions. We need to be very disciplined about any review of the assumptions—the hidden premises—on which we would have to rely in order to reach the conclusions (dire or beneficial) that get bandied about by enthusiasts on one side of the issue or the other. How likely is it that what some fear (or hope for) will come to pass? Dworkin lists other questions that have to do primarily with the slippery-slope version of the concern over the integrity of the profession. "What," he asks, "would be the social consequences of such a law? Would legally sanctioned killing make the community as a whole more callous about death?"[92] These, too, are empirical issues that cannot be settled definitively unless we conduct an actual experiment.

We need to make educated guesses, certainly. But we need also to avoid claiming more certainty than we have grounds for and to build our arguments with greater care. Above all, we need to continue trying to understand—each of us, for ourselves—both "the character of the interests people have in when and how they die" and what is meant, for instance, by "the sanctity of life." The latter phrase is frequently used in debates about abortion and euthanasia, and it is made to carry an enormous burden. Its subtlety and susceptibility to more than one interpretation are, however, underestimated. Dworkin warns that there is an underlying "confusion" about the former and "a misapprehension" about the latter.[93] I will return to consider these (and Dworkin's position on both) in Chapter 5. There, too, I will present a model of the kinds of arguments we each need to be able to make. Only with carefully constructed arguments in hand can we be confident we have adequately worked out the appropriate stance to take with our physicians.[94]

NOTES

1. William Shakespeare, *King Lear*, act 5, sc. 3, lines 314–16, in G. Blakemore Evans, ed., *The Riverside Shakespeare* (Boston: Houghton Mifflin, 1974), p. 1295.

2. See, e.g., J. Daryl Charles, "The 'Right to Die' in the Light of Contemporary Rights-Rhetoric," in John F. Kiler, Nigel M. de S. Cameron, and David L. Schiedermeyer, eds., *Bioethics and the Future of Medicine: A Christian Appraisal* (Grand Rapids, Mich.: William B. Eermans Publishing Co., 1995), pp. 263–64.

3. More than one writer has referred to what happened during that period as a "rights revolution." See, e.g., Samuel Walker, *In Defense of American Liberties: A History of the ACLU* (New York: Oxford University Press, 1990), pp. 299, 330. Lonny Shavelson, *A Chosen Death: The Dying Confront Assisted Suicide* (Berkeley: University of California Press, 1998 [New York: Simon & Schuster, 1995]), p. 151, says the current "'Rights Culture'" has seen the courts adding "a series of rights not specifically listed in [the Constitution]: women's rights, racial rights, farmworkers' rights, prisoners' rights, tenants' rights, consumers' rights, children's rights."

4. Originally printed and distributed informally, the book was first published commercially by Simon & Schuster in 1973. See "Preface," Boston Women's Health Book Collective, *Our Bodies, Ourselves: A Book By and For Women*, Revised and Expanded (New York: Simon & Schuster, 1976), 12–14, for the story of the book's development.

5. *Schloendorff v. Society of New York Hospital*, 211 N.Y. 125 (1914). See Richard E. Shugrue and Kathryn Linstromberg, "The Practitioner's Guide to Informed Consent," *Creighton Law Review* 24 (1991): 883n5.

6. *Salgo v. Leland Stanford, Jr., University Board of Trustees*, 154 Cal. App. 2d 560 (1957). See Shugrue and Linstromberg, "Informed Consent," *Creighton Law Review*: 893.

7. *Canterbury v. Spence*, 464 F.2d 772 (D.C. Cir.), cert. den., 409 U.S. 1064 (1972). See Shugrue and Linstromberg, "Informed Consent," *Creighton Law Review*: 886, 886n26.

8. Justification for taking this case—*In re Quinlan*, 70 N.J. 10 (1976) cert. den., 429 U.S. 922 (1976)—as the terminus a quo for public discussion of the right-to-die issue is given in Henry R. Glick, *The Right to Die: Policy Innovation & Its Consequences* (New York: Columbia University Press, 1992), pp. 14–15, where he documents the astonishing increase in articles on the right to die published in the immediate aftermath of *Quinlan*. See also Jeff Stryker, "Life After Quinlan," *NYT* (31 Mar. 1996): E5.

9. David J. Rothman, *Strangers at the Bedside: A History of How Law and Bioethics Transformed Medical Decision Making* (New York: Basic Books, 1991), p. 238.

10. *Cobbs v. Grant,* 8 Cal. 3d 229, 242 (1972).

11. *Barber v. Superior Court,* 147 Cal. App. 3d 1006 (1983); *Bartling v. Superior Court,* 163 Cal. App. 3d 186 (1984).

12. *Bouvia v. Superior Court,* 225 Cal. Rptr. 297 (Cal. App. 2d) (1986), at 300. The chief significance of this case is the clarification that a right to refuse treatment should not depend on the physical ability of the patient to avoid that treatment.

13. *Griswold v. Connecticut,* 381 U.S. 479, 484 (1965).

14. *Schloendorff v. Society of New York Hospital,* 211 N.Y. 125, 105 N.E. 92 (1914), at 93.

15. Judith Jarvis Thomson, *The Realm of Rights* (Cambridge, Mass.: Harvard University Press, 1990), p. 3.

16. Thomson, *Realm,* p. 69.

17. It will quickly become apparent that I strongly disagree with those who "do not think that the language and approach of rights are well suited either to sound personal decision-making or to sensible public policy" in dealing (as we so often do today) with medically managed death. See Leon R. Kass, "Is There a Right to Die?" *HCR* 23, no. 1 (Jan.- Feb. 1993): 34.

18. The subject of how and under what circumstances we waive, transfer (alienate), or forfeit our rights—and the consequences for all concerned when we do one or another of these—is a complex one, well beyond the scope of this project. For more on this subject, see Hugo Adam Bedau, "The Precarious Sovereignty of Rights," in P. Koller and K. Puhl, eds., *Currents in Political Philosophy: Justice in Social and World Order* (Vienna: Hölder-Pichler-Temsky, 1997), pp. 213–26.

19. Wesley Newcomb Hohfeld, "Some Fundamental Legal Conceptions as Applied in Judicial Reasoning," as reprinted in Walter Wheeler Cook, ed., *Fundamental Legal Conceptions,* (New Haven, Conn.: Yale University Press, 1919).

20. Alan R. White in his review of Thomson's book—*Philosophy* 66, no. 258 (Oct. 1991): 538—claims that Thomson is "completely wrong-headed, mainly owing to a disastrously uncritical acceptance of the analyses of [Hohfeld's] notions of right, claim and privilege." Neither my reading of Thomson nor the several other reviews of her book I have read have persuaded me that his radically negative assessment is on the right track.

21. Thus J. Daryl Charles is wrong when he asserts that "Every right imposes some obligations—i.e., moral demands—on others." See his "'Right to Die,'" in Kiler et al., eds., *Bioethics and the Future of Medicine,"* p. 272.

22. Thomson, *Realm,* pp. 39–43.

23. Thomson, *Realm,* p. 55 and 55n11.

24. One example of a bald statement of a right to die can be found in one of the concurring opinions in *Bouvia.* Saying that Elizabeth Bouvia had made "a conscious and informed choice that she prefers death" and that she "has an absolute right to effectuate that decision," Associate Justice Compton then went on to state that the "right to die is an integral part of our right to control our own destinies." *Bouvia v. Superior Court,* 225 Cal. Rptr. 297 (Cal. App. 2d), (1986), at 307. He proffered no explanation of this right.

25. See, e.g., Cicely Saunders and Mary Baines, *Living with Dying* (Oxford: Oxford University Press, 1983): 5; see also several pieces by Saunders cited in Ch. 2 above. Saunders and Baines are presumably among those distressed by the

affirmative conclusions John Hardwig drew in his "Is There a Duty to Die?" *HCR* 27, no. 2 (Mar.-Apr. 1997): 34–42. For a book-length discussion of the subject, see James M. Humber and Robert F. Almeder, eds., *Is There A Duty To Die?* (Totowa, N.J.: Humana Press, 2000).

26. The only other writer I have seen troubling to make this non-trivial point is columnist Ellen Goodman, who wrote, "It began with the oddest of rallying cries. People started talking about the 'right to die' as if dying were not an inevitable human condition." See her "Euthanasia as an option," *BG* (24 Apr. 1997): A27.

27. Exceptions include Ronald Dworkin's use of the phrase as a title for an article on the Supreme Court's refusal to reverse the state of Missouri's decision in the Nancy Cruzan case. See Ronald Dworkin, "The Right to Death," *The New York Review* (31 Jan. 1991): 14–17, and the title of a book edited by A. B. Downing, *Euthanasia and the Right to Death: The Case for Voluntary Euthanasia* (London: Peter Owen, 1969).

28. See, e.g., Milton D. Heifetz with Charles Mangel, *The Right to Die* (New York: Putnam's, 1975) and Glick, *Right to Die.*

29. On this undated fact sheet, that statement appears to be attributed to the Michigan State Medical Society, though no actual source is given. The address of the Hospice Federation of Massachusetts is 1420 Providence Highway, Suite 216, Norwood MA 02062.

30. See the "About NHPCO" page found at *http://www.nhpco.org/public.*

31. This is roughly the argument in *Bouvia* (1986), as we saw.

32. Thomson, *Realm,* pp. 205, 211.

33. See *Washington v. Glucksberg,* 521 U.S. 702 (1997) and *Vacco v. Quill,* 521 U.S. 793 (1997).

34. Thomson, *Realm,* p. 264 (and generally pp. 262–69).

35. Joseph Fletcher in his early and influential essay, "Euthanasia: Our Right to Die," went so far as to claim that voluntary euthanasia "is a form of suicide." See Joseph Fletcher, *Morals and Medicine* (Boston: Beacon Press, 1960 [Princeton University Press, 1954]), p. 176. He is not alone in arguing the equivalency of voluntary euthanasia and suicide. More recently, for example, Colin Brewer, proclaiming a principle he believed was "self-evident," said that the "moral issues involved in most cases of voluntary euthanasia are virtually identical to the moral issues involved in suicide." Colin Brewer, "Voluntary Euthanasia or Assisted Suicide? A Question of Freedom," *Catholic Med. Qrtrly.* 45 (Aug. 1993): 22.

36. See, e.g., Sam Howe Verhovek, "Federal Judge Stops Effort To Overturn Suicide Law," *NYT* (9 Nov. 2001): A14; "Ashcroft's Meddling," *BG* (10 Nov. 2001): A14; Betty Rollin, Barak Tulin, Faye Girsh, William S. Kilborne, Dorothy Walton (letters to the editor), "Oregon's Suicide Law, Under Siege," *NYT* (11 Nov. 2001): 12. See also Adam Liptak, "Judge Blocks U.S. Bid to Ban Suicide Law," *NYT* (18 Apr. 2002): A16. The Hemlock Society USA attacked Ashcroft in a cover story (calling him "the choice destroyer") in the inaugural issue of *End of Life Choices* 1, no. 1 (Winter 2002): 3, 15.

37. Derek Humphry and Mary Clement, *Freedom to Die: People, Politics, and the Right-to-Die Movement* (New York: St. Martin's Press, 1998), p. 117.

38. Thomson, *Realm,* p. 273–74.

39. For a discussion of the "duty to treat" in the context of AIDS, see Norman Daniels, *Seeking Fair Treatment: From the AIDS Epidemic to National Health Care Reform* (New York: Oxford University Press, 1995), pp. 13–38.

40. Thomson mentions more or less in passing that "the right to life is nowadays often said to include powers . . . as where a terminally ill patient asks to have the life-support machinery disconnected and is thought to have thereby made himself or herself no longer have a claim to not be killed" (Thomson, *Realm,* p. 285). By no means clear is whether this analysis of the right to life can withstand scrutiny, whether what is at issue in such a case really *is* a power-right, and whether—if it is one—such a power-right is a right to life rather than a right to die. Thomson does not help us out. Furthermore, I am not alone in believing that having life-saving machinery disconnected at one's request is *not* a matter of being killed.

41. I am indebted to Charles Baron for this example.

42. Philosopher Norman Daniels, for example, has made it clear in numerous conversations with me that he believes the Hohfeld-Thomson analysis is not by itself adequate to show that we do not (let alone cannot) have a claim-right to assistance with our dying.

43. One such example is the case of George Delury, who helped his wife— Myrna Lebov—end her life by giving her "a deadly dose of an antidepressant mixed with water and honey" and then pled guilty to attempted manslaughter. Delury was sentenced to six months in prison, clear evidence that his act was not deemed murder. See Garry Pierre-Pierre, "Man Who Helped Wife Die to Serve 6 Months," *NYT* (18 May 1996): 22.

44. An excellent discussion, which among other things criticizes Yale Kamisar's position that there is a moral right to die but that it should not be made a legal right, can be found in Joel Feinberg's 1991 essay, "An Unpromising Approach to the 'Right to Die,'" in his *Freedom and Fulfillment: Philosophical Essays* (Princeton, N.J.: Princeton University Press, 1992), pp. 260–82.

45. Earl Winkler, "Reflections on the State of Current Debate over Physician-Assisted Suicide and Euthanasia," *Bioethics* 9, no. 3/4 (1995): 313.

46. For further discussion, see F. M. Kamm, *Morality, Mortality,* 2 vols. (New York: Oxford University Press, 1996), vol. 2, pp. 17–140. See also Bonnie Steinbock and Alastair Norcross, eds., *Killing and Letting Die,* 2nd ed. (New York: Fordham University Press, 1994).

47. Tom L. Beauchamp and LeRoy Walters, eds., *Contemporary Issues in Bioethics,* 3rd ed. (Belmont, Calif.: Wadsworth, 1989), p. 240.

48. Christians receive no help from St. Paul. When he said "I don't accomplish the good I set out to do, and the evil I don't really want to do I find I am always doing" (Romans 7: [19]), he did not rank-order omissions and commissions; he despises equally his failure to do good on the one hand and his doing evil on the other. J. B. Phillips, trans., *The New Testament in Modern English* (New York: Macmillan, 1960), p. 330.

49. James Rachels, *The End of Life: Euthanasia and Morality* (Oxford: Oxford University Press, 1986), p. 113.

50. Rachels, *End of Life,* p. 113.

51. For further discussion, see John Ruark's "Initiating and Withdrawing Life Support: Principles and Practice in Adult Medicine," *NEJM* 318, no. 1 (7 Jan. 1988):

25–30. See also, in general, Joanne Lynn, ed., *By No Extraordinary Means* (Bloomington: Indiana University Press, 1986) and Sidney H. Wanzer, *The End of Life: How to Deal with the System, A Practical Guide for Patients and Families* (Denver, Colo.: The Hemlock Society, 2001).

52. See James Rachels, "Active and Passive Euthanasia," *NEJM* 292, no. 2 (9 Jan. 1975): 78–80, expanded in his *End of Life*, pp. 106–50.

53. Rachels, *End of Life*, p. 111.

54. Rachels, *End of Life*, pp. 148, 150.

55. Rachels, "Active and Passive Euthanasia," *NEJM*: 78; see also Rachels, *End of Life*, p. 88, and his notes, pp. 192–93, for information on the original source of the AMA statement.

56. Bonnie Steinbock, "The Intentional Termination of Life" (originally published in *Ethics in Sci. and Med.* 6, no. 1 [1979]: 59–64) and Thomas D. Sullivan, "Active and Passive Euthanasia: An Impertinent Distinction?" (originally published in *Human Life Rev.* 3, no. 3 [Summer 1977]: 40–46), reprinted in Steinbock and Norcross, eds., *Killing and Letting Die*, pp. 120–30 and 131–38, respectively.

57. Sullivan, "An Impertinent Distinction?," in Steinbock and Norcross, eds., *Killing and Letting Die*, p. 137.

58. James Rachels, "More Impertinent Distinctions and a Defense of Active Euthanasia," in Steinbock and Norcross, eds., *Killing and Letting Die*, p. 139.

59. Tom L. Beauchamp, ed., *Intending Death: The Ethics of Assisted Suicide and Euthanasia* (Upper Saddle River, N.J.: Prentice Hall, 1996).

60. David Barnard, "Ethical Issues in Hospice Care," in Denice C. Sheehan and Walter B. Forman, eds., *Hospice and Palliative Care: Concepts and Practice* (Sudbury, Mass.: Jones and Bartlett, 1996), p. 124.

61. Baruch Brody, "Withdrawal of Treatment versus Killing of Patients," in Beauchamp, ed., *Intending Death*, p. 96.

62. Judith Jarvis Thomson, "Killing and Letting Die: Some Comments," in Beauchamp, ed., *Intending Death*, pp. 104–08.

63. Alan J. Weisbard and Mark Siegler, "On Killing Patients With Kindness: An Appeal for Caution," in Lynn, ed., *By No Extraordinary Means*, p. 113.

64. Dan W. Brock, "Truth or consequences: The role of philosophers in policy-making," in his *Life and Death: Philosophical Essays in Biomedical Ethics* (Cambridge: Cambridge University Press, 1993), p. 411.

65. The roots of the doctrine are to be found "in the medieval natural law tradition, especially in the thought of Thomas Aquinas." William David Solomon, "Double Effect," in Lawrence C. Becker and Charlotte B. Becker, eds., *Encyclopedia of Ethics*, 3 vols. (New York: Routledge, 2001), vol. 1, p. 418.

66. Bruno Schüller, "The Double Effect in Catholic Thought: A Reevaluation," in Richard A. McCormick and Paul Ramsey, eds., *Doing Evil to Achieve Good: Moral Choice in Conflict Situations* (Chicago: Loyola University Press, 1978), p. 165.

67. Solomon, "Double Effect," in Becker and Becker, eds., *Encyclopedia of Ethics*, vol. 1, p. 418.

68. Schüller, "Double Effect," in McCormick and Ramsey, eds., *Doing Evil*, p. 165.

69. Philippa Foot, *Virtues and Vices* (Berkeley: University of California Press, 1978), p. 19. See also Glanville Williams, *The Sanctity of Life and the Criminal Law* (New York: Knopf, 1957), especially pp. 200–05.

70. Foot, *Virtues and Vices,* p. 20.

71. Richard A. Knox, "1 in 5 Doctors say they assisted a patient's death, survey finds," *BG* (28 Feb. 1992): 5.

72. Foot, *Virtues and Vices,* p. 20. The DDE is a piece of "dubious casuistry," according to Schüller, "Double Effect," in McCormick and Ramsey, eds., *Doing Evil,* p. 165.

73. Tim Helme, "The euthanasia debate: in reply to Lord Walton," *Jrnl. of the RSM* 89 (June 1996): 321.

74. Thomson dismantles the doctrine ("principle") of double effect, showing that the consequences of the way it handles "intent" are untenable. See her "Physician-Assisted Suicide: Two Moral Arguments," *Ethics* 109, no. 3 (Apr. 1999): 497–518.

75. See, in general, McCormick and Ramsey, eds., *Doing Evil.*

76. Sissela Bok, *Lying: Moral Choice in Public and Private Life* (New York: Pantheon Books, 1978).

77. Whatever else one might rely on to argue that occasional evildoing is permitted for a good end, it should *not* be the DDE. "The doctrine is not applied if the good effect is the result of the bad one, because that would violate the dogma that evil cannot be done that good may come." Williams, *Sanctity of Life,* p. 200.

78. Richard W. Momeyer, *Confronting Death* (Bloomington: Indiana University Press, 1988), p. 57.

79. Edith Hamilton and Huntington Cairns, eds., *Plato: The Collected Dialogues* (New York: Pantheon Books, 1961), p. 27. For an extended discussion of this matter, see Richard Kraut, *Socrates and the State* (Princeton, N.J.: Princeton University Press, 1984), pp. 3–7 and 54–90.

80. Dutch physician Pieter Admiraal, an early leader among Holland's euthanasia experts, was distressed with the first version of Oregon's "Death With Dignity" bill in part because it failed to take into account that physicians by and large do not know how to end a patient's life painlessly. "It is not so easy to kill [a patient] as you might think," he says. Pieter Admiraal, personal communication. Steven H. Miles, arguing the negative in a University of Minnesota forum titled "Should Physician Assisted Suicide be Legalized?" (in 1997) made essentially the same point. The idea that killing with morphine is easy, he said, "endlessly fascinates" only those who don't practice geriatric medicine.

81. See Luke 10: 30–37.

82. Many advocates of physician-aid-in-dying of exactly that sort turned out to want to distance themselves from Jack Kevorkian's injecting Thomas Youk with potassium chloride, which was shown on CBS's *60 Minutes,* November 22, 1998 (see Ch. 4 for further discussion). For Hemlock enthusiasts, "killing" might be thought equivalent to "speeding up the inevitable [death] with no pain"—but they might still want nothing to do with Kevorkian's activity, even though he described what he did in much the same words.

83. Fletcher, *Morals and Medicine,* p. 173. See Hilary R. Werts, "Moral Aspects of Euthanasia," *The Linacre Qrtrly.* 19, no. 2 (April 1947): 33.

84. Fletcher, *Morals and Medicine,* p. 203.

85. In a more recent (and more thorough) analysis, Franklin G. Miller and Howard Brody, "Professional Integrity and Physician-Assisted Suicide," *HCR* 25, no. 3 (May-June 1995): 8–17, reach the same conclusion as Fletcher did.

86. Ronald Dworkin, *Life's Dominion: An Argument About Abortion, Euthanasia, and Individual Freedom* (New York: Knopf, 1993), p. 182.

87. The other side of the slippery-slope issue, which I will not take up here, is that seen by the patient. There the concern is that once physician-aid-in-dying is legally permitted, patients—especially the most vulnerable ones—will be at risk. If doctors slide down the slippery slope, patients are the ones who suffer.

88. Dworkin, *Dominion*, p. 197.

89. Dworkin, *Dominion*, p. 198.

90. James Rachels insists there are two forms of the slippery-slope argument, the "logical" and the "psychological" versions, only the latter of which calls for an empirical response. (I shall return to this in Ch. 6.) Note that Rachels believes neither form of the argument provides good grounds for insisting euthanasia not be legalized. Rachels, *End of Life*, pp. 172–75.

91. Shavelson, *Chosen Death,* pp. 65, 66. Contrast this with the view of another thoughtful California physician: "It may be that society will eventually decide it wants the right to allow citizens to decide to end their lives. However, doctors *should not be partners in this.*" Lynn Sheffey, personal communication (emphasis added). The context makes clear Sheffey's concern stems not from a lack of faith in doctors, but from his belief that doctors participating in assisted death would "seriously undermine" the integrity of the medical profession.

92. Dworkin, *Dominion*, p. 182.

93. Dworkin, *Dominion*, pp. 216–17.

94. An example of a pair of arguments can be found in Thomson, "Physician-Assisted Suicide: Two Moral Arguments," *Ethics:* 497–518. The first relies on the distinction between killing and letting die, the second on the understanding that it is always (morally) impermissible for doctors to kill their patients.

4

Dealing with Death

O Lord of mysteries, how beautiful is sudden death . . .
                                                —Denise Levertov[1]

No single individual or event can be credited with having made "death and dying" the common and controversial topic it had become by the end of the twentieth century. Evidence that more than one of the related issues has caught public attention comes in many forms. One dramatic example is the nineteen-segment program on "The End of Life: Exploring Death in America," which aired on National Public Radio (NPR) between November 1997 and April 1998.[2] An even more startling contribution appeared on the "Living Arts" pages of the *Boston Globe* some three years earlier. Morris Schwartz, a sociology professor at Brandeis University, was "teaching his final class . . . on a subject of unusual intimacy: his approaching death." The article took up two-thirds of the section's front page, plus another entire page. The story's subhead set the tone: "Facing a fatal disease, Morris Schwartz teaches how to live until the last moment."[3] Less than a week later, the *Globe* carried a letter in response[4] and—when Schwartz died nine months afterwards—in addition to a lengthy obituary ran an editorial on his death and published yet another letter.[5] Then, when a former student of Schwartz's who had visited him weekly during the final months of his life published a book with an intimate portrayal of those meetings,[6] the *Globe* reviewed it as well.[7] This extraordinary amount of coverage to the final days of one man, who prior to his dying was well known to other sociologists and his many former students but not to the general population of Greater Boston, is a strong indication that the newspaper's editors believe people are fascinated with reflections on dying. Clearly, writing and talking about experiences connected with death are not considered in poor taste today. Editors of many publications seem ready, perhaps even eager, to provide a forum.

Around the same time, another story had appeared, similar in the extent to which its central feature was the experience of death, but providing an even clearer sign of changing times. This was the case of "futurist" Tom Mandel, who shared "on-line, with a wide audience, his own experience of dying." Mandel was "one of the first (if not the first)" to do so.[8] That more would follow as cyberspace expanded to fill the interstices of our lives (and, apparently, deaths) is hardly surprising; two deaths late in the year 2000, in places as far removed from each other as Wichita, Kansas, and Shanghai, are cases in point.[9]

Before turning to explore three of the most important possible approaches to dealing with dying, I will set the stage by reviewing three very different accounts of women who died under (to one degree or another) a physician's watchful eye. The story of Janet Adkins (in 1990) moved from the daily papers—where it attracted considerable attention and began the process that has made the name "Jack Kevorkian" so familiar—to become a subject of discussion in the professional journals. The short unhappy story of "Debbie" appeared anonymously in *JAMA* (in 1988) and set off a firestorm of debate in that journal and elsewhere within medical professional circles. Much more fully formed is the story of Diane, a woman in Rochester, New York, whose physician—Timothy Quill—helped her end her life. Immediately after his account appeared in the pages of the *NEJM* (in 1991), debates about the story leapt to the popular press and back to professional journals.

Janet Adkins, an Oregon woman in her early fifties who had been diagnosed with Alzheimer's disease, became—on June 4, 1990—the first of more than 130 individuals whom the retired Michigan pathologist, Dr. Jack Kevorkian, eventually helped to die. Kevorkian himself tells the story in his book, *Prescription: Medicide,* giving a reasonably full report of what transpired, though cautious readers will want to check other sources for more objective versions.[10] Indeed, Kevorkian devotes much of the chapter in question to letting the reader know what steps he personally took to assure that he had handled everything with as much careful attention to every detail as one could possibly have hoped for. The focus is on him at least as much as it is on Janet Adkins and her plight. Moreover, Kevorkian also managed (in a single sentence) to slide over the issue that was most troubling to those who knew, or soon learned, what he had done: Janet Adkins was not, by standard measures, terminally ill. "Even though from a physical stand point Janet was not imminently terminal," he conceded, "there seemed little doubt that mentally she was." And that was enough for him. In the minds of many (including those most sympathetic to the idea of physician-aid-in-dying), that meant she was not the right person for this kind of physician assistance. Kevorkian, however, was dismissive of any such concerns: "I decided to accept her as the first candidate—a qualified, justifiable candidate if not 'ideal.'" He was not worried, he said, about his "vulnerability to criticism of picayune and overly emotional critics."[11]

The fact that Janet Adkins was not terminally ill, though hardly the only issue, was central to the controversy aroused by her death and the manner in which it was brought about. "For months, lawyers and ethics experts have debated the morality of a makeshift device built by Dr. Jack Kevorkian to help terminally ill people kill themselves," we are told in an article that appeared six months after Adkins's death, when Kevorkian was in court for the first time. "The ensuing debate over Mrs. Adkins's death led to a seizure of the device [Kevorkian dubbed it a "Mercitron"] by the authorities, [and] a temporary injunction banning its use." Murder charges were brought against Kevorkian but later dropped.[12] No one really knew what to do about him.

In the meantime, however, those interested in physician-assisted suicide had all learned the name "Janet Adkins." The lines were drawn sharply: Either she was an innocent dupe to be pitied, or she was a pioneer helping blaze a trail to a new territory where freedom to decide the time and manner of one's death would be the norm. Her case would continue to be discussed, as the number of Kevorkian's patients—or victims, depending on one's point of view—increased. She came to symbolize for many the possibility that help might be available outside the world of mainstream medicine, which seemed to be dragging its feet in typically conservative fashion.

"Debbie" had appeared on the scene two years earlier, but the story of this woman (whoever she was) made its splash in the medical rather than the popular press.[13] An anonymous submission to *JAMA* of fewer than 600 words, it is a first-person account of a middle-of-the-night visit by the medical resident on duty to a dying patient on a gynecologic-oncology unit. Briefly, what happened was this: The resident, after a quick glance at the woman's chart and an update from the nurse, chose to respond to the patient's plea to "get this over with" (which is all she said to him) by giving her a lethal dose of morphine. The woman with her at the time, presumably her mother, said nothing. So here we have a doctor simply deciding, essentially on the spur of the moment and with no consultation, to end the life of a patient he has never seen before. If the story was true (nothing in succeeding issues of the journal suggested any reason to doubt its accuracy), it symbolized in dramatic fashion exactly what those opposed to physician assistance in dying—including doctors themselves—fear most. Doctors, given the opportunity, will make arbitrary decisions about who should live and who should die. Quite likely they will sometimes do so for the wrong reasons, with too little information and without consultation, with no controls or checks and balances on their behavior.

A heated debate followed, including over whether the journal had any business publishing such a piece (particularly anonymously) at all. In addition to a raft of letters arguing virtually every angle of the story's implications, two essays and an explanatory editorial appeared a few weeks later. The first paragraph of the opening commentary, "Doctors Must Not Kill," ended with an appalled "What in the world is going on?" Later in the essay came a veritable trumpet blast: "These are perilous times for our profession." The closing exhortation by then could have been predicted: "Now is not the time for promoting neutral discussion. Rather, now is the time for the medical profession to rally in defense of its fundamental moral principles, to repudiate any and all acts of direct and intentional killing by physicians." The essay was signed by four physicians known nationally for their opposition to physician-aid-in-dying.[14]

A much more balanced and calmer essay followed. In "Debbie's Dying: Mercy Killing and the Good Death," the author agreed that "what (apparently) transpired that night was unconscionable. . . . The whole process, from beginning to end, was morally unacceptable." He goes on, however, to draw lessons from "this ambiguous and melodramatic diary." Pointing out that although "the outrage of Debbie's death reminds us that we must never abandon the cardinal purpose of medical care—to save and sustain life and never intentionally to harm or kill," there is also a second lesson. And that lesson is "that we must not destroy the virtue of that commitment by using medical art to prolong dying and puritanically refuse to relieve suffering."[15]

The sharp divide in the debate evidenced by the letters—eighteen of which were published (out of the 150 received)—is indicative of how troubling the subject is for the medical profession.[16] All the more reason for patients and doctors to talk about their respective views, as Sidney Wanzer (among others) has urged. (I will return to this topic in the next chapter.) The strength of the feeling expressed and the potency of (some of) the arguments surely vindicate the decision to publish the anonymous piece in the first place. The editor, George Lundberg, explained: "We published 'It's Over, Debbie' to provoke responsible debate within the medical profession and by the public about euthanasia in the United States in 1988." He ended by saying that publishing the anonymous essay was a way for the journal to demonstrate "its belief that the ethics of euthanasia must be debated anew."[17] His position seems more constructive than that taken by the doctors who insisted it was "not the time for promoting neutral discussion." If not then, when?

The third woman whose story helped stir a public debate over physician-aid-in-dying in a very personal way was Diane. The contrast between the 1991 *NEJM* essay written by her internist, Dr. Timothy Quill—"A Case of

Individualized Decision Making"[18]—and the anonymous "Debbie" piece three years earlier could hardly have been greater. First, Quill signed his article, acknowledging publicly that he had done what he knew many commentators would criticize as not only illegal but also immoral (and in direct conflict with the much-vaunted "integrity of the profession"). Second, his article was some 2,500 words long, giving him space to anticipate questions and provide answers of the sort denied to thoughtful readers of the "Debbie" essay. Third, and most important, Diane was a patient whom Quill had known well over a period of years. As he made eminently clear in the article, his decision to give her a prescription for barbiturates that he knew she intended to use to commit suicide was made only after long and careful discussions with her. "I wrote the prescription with an uneasy feeling about the boundaries I was exploring—spiritual, legal, professional, and personal," Quill told his readers. "Yet I also felt strongly that I was setting her free to get the most out of the time she had left, and to maintain dignity and control on her own terms until her death."[19]

Among the concerns that Quill's article raised was his acknowledged willingness to fudge facts. When Diane died, her husband phoned Quill, who went to the house. "I called the medical examiner to inform him that a hospice patient had died. When asked about the cause of death, I said, 'acute leukemia.' . . . Although acute leukemia was the truth, it was not the whole story."[20] Yet that was surely also only a minor wrinkle in the overall fabric. The far knottier concerns were whether a doctor should knowingly and deliberately help a patient die and what limitations there should be on such help. For Quill himself, it is clear from his published account of the experience, a thread of considerable importance in holding it all together was the long-standing doctor-patient relationship. "Diane taught me about the range of help I can provide *if I know people well* and if I allow them to say what they really want. . . . She taught me that I can take small risks *for people that I really know and care about*."[21]

Almost lost in the uproar caused by Quill's article was a sentence of utmost importance, one that gives a strong hint about how unfinished the whole debate is. "I wonder," he wrote in his closing paragraph, "how many families and physicians secretly help patients over the edge into death in the face of such severe suffering."[22] We all need to remember that questions about whether physician-aid-in-dying should be legalized are by no means the only ones to be asked, important though they are. In the end, what can and will be done by physicians, with and for their dying patients, will almost certainly remain a very personal matter between the two principals.

In the meantime, Quill's experience is instructive. This is not the place to go into the details of what Quill himself wryly calls his "legal difficulties."[23] It should be noted, however, that giving what he truly believed was the best possible care for one of his dying patients (and then sharing his struggle over his decision with the world) took a kind of courage we do not typically expect our physicians will need to exercise. Quill has admitted that, despite his careful consideration of the steps he was taking, he did not fully appreciate what he was getting into. "After the article was published, I received an unwanted education as to how our legal system both works and doesn't work, and how it is influenced by political forces. Although I intended to challenge the profession of medicine, I underestimated the extent to which the general public and the legal system would become interested and involved." Criminal charges against him were considered, ranging from "tampering with public records to manslaughter." When the case was presented to a grand jury, however, it was determined that his "actions did not warrant prosecution. The New York State Health Department also reviewed the case; it subsequently found no evidence of professional misconduct."[24] From the outset, "family, close friends, patients, practice partners, colleagues, office staff, and staff at the Genesee Hospital" supported him. The "leadership within the American College of Physicians and the Society of General Internal Medicine took the risk of expressing public support when there was doubt about the outcome of the grand jury investigation."[25]

The stories of Janet Adkins, "Debbie," and Diane show that strong feelings and disagreements dominate the ongoing debate over physician-aid-in-dying. Moreover, these stories both reflect and elicit three very particular issues: Can doctors be controlled (Kevorkian the freelancer proved very difficult to "control") if physician-aid-in-dying is not legalized? Would legalizing physician-aid-in-dying lead to abuse (that is, even more cases—implicitly condoned—of the "Debbie" variety) or is legalization the best way to control a practice good doctors will engage in anyway? And, finally, should physician-aid-in-dying be legalized because that would mean the Quills of the world would not have to struggle so long and so privately with their consciences and would not have to risk untoward legal consequences of what they judge to be appropriate end-of-life care? With these questions in mind, let's look now at three kinds of help that loom on the horizon as at least theoretical possibilities for those of us concerned about how we will die.

DO-IT-YOURSELF HELP

In the United States, the most basic of the questions about how we want to or should die have been thrust before us in recent years in large part thanks to the repeated headlines generated by the activities of Dr. Jack Kevorkian. His invention of a "suicide machine" several years ago, it has been said, helped "set the stage for a national debate on physician-assisted suicide."[26] On the one hand, even as public uneasiness with his behavior grew, a parade of individuals continued to seek him out for the particular form of assistance he offered. Media reaction to the many deaths—perhaps especially to the non-terminal patients he helped die—was largely negative.[27] On the other hand, from the outset there was obvious support for what Kevorkian was doing, and many have clearly seen him as "a strange-but-good-hearted crusader."[28] Certainly he deserves credit for having forced the issue onto the public agenda; for years, it was not possible to read the daily papers regularly and escape word of Jack Kevorkian's crusade to help people die when they wanted to.[29]

The great American love affair with quick and easy solutions to every problem—living in a push-button society has encouraged us more than ever to seek instant gratification—seems to resonate with Kevorkian's willingness to help people die with few questions asked and essentially no waiting period required. Surely this "quick-fix" aspect of Kevorkian's procedure was part of the appeal his "suicide machine" had for those who saw themselves in desperate straits, wanting to end their lives but not knowing how (or being able) to do so on their own.

Such a benefit may be more illusory, more purely psychological, than actual. Not everyone agrees that weighty matters of life and death should be decided and dealt with quickly if they do not have to be. A detailed story Lonny Shavelson tells in his book, *A Chosen Death: The Dying Confront Assisted Suicide,* helps illuminate the disadvantages of what he calls "Freelance Euthanasia."[30] Still, in a day when anyone who reads the newspaper knows that physician-assisted suicide is not legal in this country, too few have the kind of close and well-established relationship with their doctors that Timothy Quill describes having had with Diane. The drawing power of someone like Kevorkian, who repeatedly demonstrated his willingness to bring relief to dying persons bold enough to seek him out, should not surprise us. Many reasoned that although it was perhaps a nuisance to go to Michigan, at least the desired help would be forthcoming. Legal and other problems no doubt seemed eminently manageable, not least because Kevorkian was so frequently acquitted of charges against him.[31]

Far more important than sheer availability (which in any case applied only to "those few who can make their way to Michigan and are willing to join a macabre sideshow"[32]) is something else that even Kevorkian's opponents are willing to acknowledge he has accomplished. By campaigning for public acceptance of physician-assisted suicide as no one else had, he made the rights and wrongs of physician-aid-in-dying a matter for public discussion. Derek Humphry, for example, while acknowledging that Kevorkian "muddied the waters," also says he "injected life and action into the smoldering [right to die] movement," and that his "essential contribution to the right-to-die movement was the enormous scope of the publicity."[33] Timothy Quill likewise credits Kevorkian with having helped press the debate forward and having marked its extremes. His contribution, Quill says, is to have "defined the margins" and "galvanized public awareness," to have been a "provocateur beyond belief."[34] Even in the midst of criticizing the extreme behavior ("Jack Kevorkian is on a rampage"; "Dr. Kevorkian is out of control"), Quill and his co-author in a *New York Times* op-ed piece, Betty Rollin, reminded their readers that "Dr. Kevorkian's early actions served an important purpose. He forced Americans to acknowledge the intolerable suffering of the terminally ill and helped challenge government and medicine to find better ways to help them."[35] In the *Boston Globe,* on the fifth anniversary of Kevorkian's first assisted death, Jack Lessenberry repeatedly commented on the crucial role the man from Michigan had played. "In 5 years, [a] once-obscure physician has made assisted suicide a national issue," and "the man who built the suicide machine is possibly the best-known—and most controversial—physician in the nation," Lessenberry wrote; "his actions have dramatically focused attention on what are usually called 'right-to-die' issues."[36]

Others, too, have argued that Kevorkian's activities have had benefits. The Sovereign Foundation, a "private foundation . . . committed to the belief that people thrive to the extent that they control their own destiny," gave its 1995 annual award to Kevorkian.[37] A group called "Physicians for Mercy" (based, perhaps significantly, in Kevorkian's home state of Michigan), made news when it offered Kevorkian "some organized support" (the first such offer since he began his "crusade") by "proposing 10 guidelines that they hoped would win acceptance for the practice by regulating it."[38] More surprising was the report that the *BMJ* in London had declared Kevorkian a "hero," praising him for his courage.[39] Frank A. Oski, a physician, had insisted already in 1994 that "Dr. Jack Kevorkian should be regarded as a hero,"[40] and a year later, Greg Pence (writing in a British journal, aiming to explain attitudes in the United States toward Kevorkian) wrote that "[a]mong ordinary Americans, Kevorkian is approaching the status of a folk-hero."[41]

Most of the praise for Kevorkian, however, as one would expect, has come from those who sought and received his help, or from their surviving friends and family. Because Kevorkian himself was the source of the story that his first patient, Janet Adkins, opened her eyes one last time after activating the "Mercitron" and said, "Thank you, thank you," some have been skeptical about her expressed gratitude.[42] But there are other examples—such as the videotape made by a Canadian whom Kevorkian helped to die (in Detroit), which was played for reporters after the death. In it, the man is said to have "praised Dr. Kevorkian as 'a most courageous and often misunderstood physician.'"[43] More impressive yet, for some, are testimonials by such sober-minded citizens as Bradford Washburn, longtime director of Boston's Museum of Science. "I am amazed by the furor caused by Dr. Jack Kevorkian's extraordinary services to those in agony or misery near the end of their lives. . . . Our laws in this regard are as intolerable as the pain," he wrote in a presumably unsolicited letter to the editor of the *Boston Globe*.[44]

There are, however, numerous very legitimate objections to Kevorkian's relentless campaign to make physician-assisted suicide available essentially on demand. Most of the concerns take one of two forms, both connected with Kevorkian's status as a freelancer. The first, though troubling, might almost be dismissed as trivial; the second is complex and extremely serious.

The trivial matter has to do with Kevorkian's suicide machine itself. Although the instinctive reaction of many Americans is to admire someone who can invent a piece of equipment that will do a particular job, the result in Kevorkian's case is that his various devices have a bit too much of Rube Goldberg about them.[45] By his own admission, his first "Mercitron" was put together not quite with duct tape and baling wire, but with oddments he picked up at flea markets, garage sales, and out of his own "accumulated pile of useless junk."[46] The idea that one's exit from the world is to be facilitated by such a makeshift gadget may be troubling—particularly to those already distressed by too great a reliance at the other extreme on gleamingly new, high-tech medical equipment.

The ways Kevorkian presented himself and the role he carved out for himself were more important factors. Many who might have been inclined to support his efforts were alienated by his personality, by the extreme position he took, and by the way he promoted his cause (and himself). I will examine these personal aspects of the story in my Profile of him, below. Here it will suffice to look briefly at the many ways Kevorkian's behavior falls short of what received opinion tells us a doctor's behavior should be. What he has done utterly fails to fit the criteria most serious commentators on doctor-patient relations recommend, most especially when it comes to care for the dying.

Among those who have been quoted criticizing Kevorkian for helping end the lives of patients with whom he has had "no long-term doctor patient relationship" is, not surprisingly, Timothy Quill.[47] But of course that problem is not unique to patients dying with Kevorkian's help. In *Parade Magazine*, former Surgeon General C. Everett Koop was once quoted saying that one of the "great problems in our mobile society has to do with the decisions at the end of life. . . . It used to be that your doctor knew you. Now you die at the hands of someone you never saw before."[48]

Part of what unsettles us is that matters of life and death—literally— need the most thoughtful and careful discussion imaginable; this is difficult to arrange in haste or with persons (perhaps especially doctors) whom we do not know well. Even if it is granted that Kevorkian typically met both with those who sought his help and with members of their families, and that he discussed at least some of their other options, additional concerns have surrounded his activities. Kevorkian is a pathologist, not a psychiatrist trained to understand and help others sort out their feelings; neither is he an internist, trained to understand the somatic distresses of living patients. The argument is difficult to dismiss that he is not competent to judge either when a person is ready to die or when a person's other options have been exhausted.

Then there is the plain and simple sentiment that doctors should not kill. If there is room for debate about whether the physician-assisted death that Diane received with Timothy Quill's help counts as "killing," there was much less about what Kevorkian was doing. And once CBS showed a videotape of him actually injecting lethal drugs into a patient named Thomas Youk, most viewers seemed convinced there was no longer any question; they found it difficult to understand that action as anything other than direct killing.[49] Kevorkian appeared to many, at least in this case, to have violated the particular rules that should govern personal encounters between doctors and their patients as well as the general rules of the profession. The "integrity of the profession" argument loomed large against him.

The fact that Kevorkian also worked completely on his own made people nervous. Other doctors neither chose to assist him nor to imitate him, and no other physicians (as far as we know) have built their own version of the "Mercitron." If he really was right, one might wonder, why didn't others follow suit? Kevorkian ran a one-man show, where he operated as producer, director, and star performer. The only thing he didn't do, his opponents would say, is take his vaudeville show on the road.[50] Seeking no approval but his own self-assured conviction that he had right on his side, Kevorkian was the ultimate freelancer; he threatened to capsize the whole ship of hope known as "physician-aid-in-dying."[51] The major concerns about Kevorkian's behavior have been listed thus: the possibility (even likelihood) of "abuse, lack of social control, physicians acting without accountability, and unverifiable circumstances of a patient's death."[52]

Finally, a little-discussed feature of the Kevorkian story is one that becomes visually apparent to anyone who reviews media reports of his activities. The vast majority of the articles and the bulk of the discussion have always had to do with how to handle Kevorkian, legally—whether and how he was to be charged, how he responded to indictments, how his lawyers addressed the prosecution's own provocative attacks, what juries decided. The issue thus became, to an unfortunate degree, one of what to do about Kevorkian rather than the more important matter of what physicians ought to do for their dying patients. The need for serious discussion of the morality of physician-aid-in-dying continued; Kevorkian became a distraction, steadily more of a sideshow. He was so far away from the mainstream that any residual benefits from his activities had to be seen merely in terms of the very personal benefit (if that is what it is) to the persons he helped to die. That is not nothing, of course, especially for the patient who has found the desired relief with Kevorkian's help. But it does not advance our understanding of the moral issues, and it does not help those who (for whatever reason) have not been ready or willing or able to turn to Kevorkian for help.

PROFILE: JACK KEVORKIAN

Sometimes things work out for the best. When I told people I was writing about physician-assisted dying, even before they knew I intended to interview key figures in the ongoing debate, most would respond with a salacious smirk, "Oh, so you're going to see Kevorkian." I would then confess that although I thought I really ought to talk to the man, I had no desire to meet him. Nothing I had read about or by him gave me reason to think I wanted to travel to Michigan simply for the opportunity to meet in person this odd purveyor of death.

Nonetheless, I dutifully wrote to his lawyer seeking an interview. To say I was relieved when I got a brisk note back simply stating "Dr. Kevorkian does not give interviews" is probably an understatement.[53] But I was also surprised. My very fat folder of clippings on Jack Kevorkian and his latest doings, and the number of articles in professional journals discussing and dissecting his activities, had me assuming this media-hound would be delighted to have one more person express an interest in what he had been up to since Janet Adkins's death in 1990. But Dr. Kevorkian wouldn't see me. Despite never meeting him, however, I—like most other Americans who read the papers—know a great deal about him.

An additional clue to the sort of person Jack Kevorkian really is comes in his book, provocatively titled *Prescription: Medicide*. But those who expect the book (which appeared shortly after Kevorkian helped Janet Adkins die) to be aimed primarily at explaining the author's position on physician-aid-in-dying are in for a surprise. Fully the first three-quarters of the volume is devoted instead to his long-standing and rather peculiar ideas about the potential benefits of doing medical experiments on death-row prisoners.[54] Almost regardless of their views on capital punishment, readers are likely to come away from reading this tale of Kevorkian's growing obsession with their own growing uneasiness. Kevorkian is truly out on a limb by himself on this matter. He slips with startling rapidity from discussing why death-row inmates should be allowed to choose death by lethal injection in order that they might donate their organs for organ-transplant purposes to his conviction that "the wellspring of morality is the mores of a people." Then, in the space of three pages, he moves to a discussion of birth control and euthanasia. At the very least, this is a remarkable progression of thought (which can hardly be dignified with the word "argument").[55] With that, however, he is at last off and running (in the final four of his seventeen chapters) on the campaign to convince the world that patients should have access to death on demand from their doctors.

Some portions of what Kevorkian reports about the history of medical experimentation are both interesting and accurate.[56] Nonetheless, confidence in his abilities as a scholar fades quickly. Two instances of what must be deliberate distortion (a failure to grasp the significance of what he had read would have been bad enough) in matters closer to the subject under discussion here will suffice to show why. When he wrote that "[m]ercy killings are on the increase. More and more doctors openly admit to having secretly helped suffering patients die," I turned eagerly to his footnote to see how he documented this "fact."[57] His evidence, it turns out, is the single piece written by Timothy Quill about a single case—which, incidentally, Quill never refers to as a "mercy killing."[58] Then Kevorkian begins the next chapter by discussing the "proclamation by a special medical panel . . . that it is ethical for doctors to help terminal patients commit suicide," which he says he saw as "a milestone breakthrough." Neither the article he cited nor its predecessor is a "proclamation" as we normally use that word.[59]

Three final points about Kevorkian: First, when assisted suicide is on the agenda, Kevorkian himself as often as not becomes the subject of the discussion. A case in point is the book *Doctor Assisted Suicide and the Euthanasia Movement* (1994), in which chapters on such broad topics as "Euthanasia in The Netherlands" and "Physician-Assisted Suicide: Ideas in Conflict" are preceded by a chapter devoted narrowly to "Dr. Kevorkian and Assisted Suicide."[60] That *Time* magazine should have an article on Kevorkian in late 1991, when he was just hitting his stride, is not surprising; that piece was later reprinted in a textbook on moral controversies.[61] More recently, Marilyn Webb—in her 1997 book *The Good Death* (written for a general audience)—also felt constrained to discuss Kevorkian. Numerous miscellaneous references are supplemented by an entire chapter, "Dr. Kevorkian's Challenge: Two Deaths in Michigan."[62]

Second, Kevorkian's flamboyant style—his outbursts and antics—has fueled headlines, threatening to turn the whole matter into a serialized soap opera starring Jack Kevorkian. Never mind that editors have sometimes quite gratuitously used a picture of Kevorkian's gadgetry (with or without its operator) to accompany serious articles about physician-aid-in-dying.[63] Other illustrations have been less sober. Once we were treated to a photo of Kevorkian burning a "cease and desist" order from Michigan regulators (demanding that he "stop practicing medicine"), with the jocular caption "Heated response."[64] On an earlier occasion, Kevorkian dressed up as Thomas Jefferson, claiming Jefferson as his legitimate predecessor. He gave reporters "what he said was the text of an 1813 letter in which Thomas Jefferson discusses the advantages of developing a preparation from poisonous plants that could be used to end life painlessly."[65] Another time Kevorkian was pictured in (cardboard) stocks; that time he declared the trial against him "was a throwback to the Middle Ages."[66] Then there were the times it was Kevorkian's own extreme language that garnered headlines: "Kevorkian sees role as just 'executioner'" and "Kevorkian Repeatedly Disrupts His Trial, Calling It a Lynching" are but two examples.[67]

Last, and most disturbing, is the way Kevorkian has set himself up as the arbiter of what is right and proper. A *New York Times* article (for which Kevorkian refused to be interviewed) carried the subhead "For Kevorkian, Rules Are His Own"; his feisty lawyer Geoffrey Fieger (also no slouch at generating headlines[68]) was quoted saying that his client "hates authority figures." The reporter continues, calling attention among other things to Kevorkian's extreme language: "Yet the doctor is himself by all accounts overbearing and contemptuous of anyone who disagrees with him, calling his critics 'Nazis,' 'eunuchs,' and 'mental cripples.'"[69] For such a man to decide, unilaterally, that he is the one to force the issue—and then for him to proceed to try to do so—is insulting to the serious and thoughtful commentators who have struggled with the subject of physician-aid-in-dying for so long. "CBS said Dr. Kevorkian had told Mr. [Mike] Wallace that he wanted to force a trial on euthanasia charges in the hope that it would fail and set a legal precedent," one account prior to the public showing of the videotape of Youk's death reported.[70] In the aftermath of the showing, one writer said that "the grisly logic is at last laid bare," and then proceeded to join numerous others who quoted Kevorkian's remark that the "issue's got to be raised to the level where it is finally decided."[71] Why precisely now? "I am tired of all the hypocrisy," Kevorkian was quoted in another article as having said, "and we're going to end this, one way or another."[72] My own observations, made at the time, included this:

Jack Kevorkian gave no explanation on this [*60 Minutes*] program (nor has he in the past) of why we should welcome him as the self-appointed guardian of our rights. In the end, he admitted—tellingly—that he was doing all of this for himself. Why we should accept Kevorkian's version of the issue, namely that the right to end one's own life is the ultimate in "self-determination," is now less clear than ever. . . . From here on, this particular discussion is about Kevorkian, not about society as a whole.[73]

Kevorkian may have helped "galvanize the public" as Quill puts it; he may have turned the physician-aid-in-dying discussion into one that can be debated across socio-economic and intellectual barriers, as Humphry stresses. But Kevorkian has utterly failed to provide us with evidence that *he* should be the one to determine policy. We need to think about what he has done and what he has said, yes—but we need to realize that is not the end of the story. Kevorkian having been sentenced to prison following his conviction in the Youk case is only one piece of evidence of this truth. Even though "his public voice has been muted," analyses of those who died with Kevorkian's assistance continue to be made. Whether these studies will significantly alter anyone's view of Kevorkian is doubtful.[74]

LEGAL HELP

The social issues surrounding physician-aid-in-dying and the vigorous public discourse (the shape of which has been so dramatically affected by Kevorkian, among others) have played a major role in turning the whole matter into one for the ballot box and the courts. The anxieties raised by the "Debbie" story seem, in the minds of some, to connect with the current state of affairs in Holland. Euthanasia in Holland is an enormous subject on its own, and this is not the place to discuss it in detail. I will focus only on why Holland continues to be held up by many in the United States and elsewhere as a model. (Whether it is a model for ill or for good is controversial, depending on how observers view the situation in the Netherlands.) First, however, a few words about the vast and complex subject of the current legal status of physician-aid-in-dying in the United States (and how we arrived at this point), will serve as a preface to the discussion of the Dutch "model" and its possible relevance for the United States.

In the United States today, active euthanasia (whether it is considered "killing"—"mercy" or otherwise) is illegal. On the other hand, although assisting a suicide is illegal in thirty-five states, there are fifteen where it is not prohibited by law.[75] Knowing what the law says does not by itself settle what anyone *ought* to do, however, unless obedience to the law is seen as the prime value; others may believe that their conscientious commitment to a higher moral principle permits exceptions.

The first flares were lit on the West Coast in the early 1990s. The state of Washington (in 1991) and then California (in 1992) narrowly defeated legislation that would have legalized euthanasia. I have already referred (in Chapter 1) to the scathing criticism of the role played by the Catholic church in the California fight, in particular. Ronald Dworkin makes the point as well, also explicitly identifying the Hemlock Society as one of the groups that lobbied for passage of these two bills.[76]

A subsequent fight in Oregon went rather differently, following an unusual and convoluted path to ultimate success (not to say vindication) for the proponents of legalized assistance in dying. In November 1994, the Oregon "Death With Dignity Act" (Ballot Measure 16) was passed by the narrowest of margins—51 percent to 49 percent.[77] Promptly challenged, it was struck down in federal district court in August 1995.[78] The Act was eventually re-instated when the Circuit Court of Appeals overturned the judge's decision in February 1997, ruling that the opponents did not have standing; the Supreme Court refused to grant certiorari (that is, would not hear arguments on it).[79] Undeterred, opponents persuaded the Oregon legislature to send Measure 16 back to the voters, where it appeared on the ballot in November 1997 (without changes) as Ballot Measure 51.[80] The effort to engineer a rejection of the bill the second time around was a dismal failure; the measure passed decisively. The significance was not lost on commentators. As one of them put it: "The professional landscape of medicine changed irrevocably on 4 November 1997 when Oregon voters decided by a 60 percent to 40 percent margin to oppose repeal of the state's Death with Dignity Act."[81] The passage of Measure 51 did not bring an immediate end to the legal skirmishing, however. Only in 1998 did the legal dust begin to settle.[82]

Starting at that point, we finally have on native soil a "laboratory" where we can begin to study what the availability of legal physician-aid-in-dying means for medical practitioners and patients alike.[83] Immediately it was clear there would be no wild stampede among dying patients to get help from their physicians. Four months after the bill was passed, Timothy Egan wrote in the *New York Times*: "No One Rushing in Oregon To Use a New Suicide Law: Doctors and Pharmacists Ponder Their Role," though less than two weeks later there was a death to report.[84] Another five months passed before statistics were released, at which point it became official news that no great landslide down the infamous slippery slope had taken place. (Spokesmen for the Catholic church nonetheless, predictably, expressed great sorrow over these few deaths.) A total of ten patients had taken advantage of the new law to obtain legally prescribed lethal drugs; only eight had died using the drugs, however (two died of natural causes without taking the drugs).[85] Even after a full year in force, the nation's only assisted-suicide law had been used to end the lives of barely more than a dozen (fifteen) terminally ill patients.[86] Later, in a newspaper report on the *NEJM* article published at the one-year point, Oregon health officials were said to have found that "fears that the law would be used as an easy way out by people afraid of financial ruin or extreme pain proved unfounded."[87]

The authors of a formal study (carried out in 1999) of Oregon's experience with the law concluded their report with this observation: "Many people feared that if physician-assisted suicide was legalized, it would be disproportionately chosen by or forced on terminally ill patients who were poor, uneducated, uninsured, or fearful of the financial consequences of their illness," but the researchers found "no evidence to support these fears."[88] In other words, passage of the Oregon Death with Dignity Act

(ODDA) in 1997 has not led to swarms of people fleeing to Oregon to die. A further report, published by the Oregon Death With Dignity Legal Defense and Education Center on the third anniversary of the law's implementation, concluded: "Two years of statistics from the Oregon Health Division reveal the law is a thoughtful and well-crafted piece of legislation. Moreover, the law is seldom used by terminally ill individuals facing difficult deaths. Rather, the law exists as one option along the continuum of care and provides great comfort to those in need."[89] These remarks are fully consonant with the results of a survey of physicians' actual experience with ODDA, reported earlier in 2000 by Linda Ganzini, an associate professor at Oregon Health Sciences University (OHSU) and a faculty scholar of the Open Society Institute's Project on Death in America.[90]

Still more recent research was reported by Ganzini at a conference ("Physician Assisted Dying: Assessing the State of the Debate," sponsored by the University of Minnesota Center for Bioethics) in April 2001 and published a month later. As a follow-up to the earlier study, qualitative interviews were conducted with thirty-five physicians who had actually written prescriptions for lethal drugs under ODDA. It appears that doctors who have received requests for assistance with suicide have found care for the terminally ill more intellectually satisfying than other doctors have. Furthermore, these physicians did more to increase their knowledge of palliative care than did doctors who received no requests for lethal prescriptions.

Most striking is the finding that prior to receiving requests for help with dying, details of the law were uppermost in physicians' minds, whereas when requests actually came, the emotional impact of dealing with the request became central. Great intimacy with the dying patient developed in these cases. Above all, doctors sought confidence that the request was congruent with the patient's overall life. Further indications that we will not soon see medical killing fields in Oregon as a result of ODDA is the report that doctors found the experience of dealing with a request for assistance stressful, making them dread the next request. Helping someone commit suicide does not, according to this study, get easier—nor does legalized assisted suicide undermine attempts to improve care for dying patients.[91]

What conclusions are to be drawn from the experience in Oregon? Even though the "Death With Dignity" law has been in effect several years now, it is still in its early days. Nonetheless, cautious optimism about this first natural laboratory is beginning to be expressed. Timothy Quill, for example, saying first that of course we still don't know how the story in Oregon is going to turn out, went on to mention several shifts in care for the dying that have taken place in Oregon since the law went into effect and that may be a direct result of ODDA. Certainly they are steps in the right direction. "The preliminary data are good," he insisted. There have been few cases of doctors helping patients die, the number of prescriptions for morphine has increased, doctors as well as nurses are attending palliative care conferences, referrals to Hospice are up, and managed care organizations are competing over who gives the best end-of-life care. The whole process seems to have been opened up; the discussion has now been moved "over ground instead of underground."[92] Supporting much of what Quill observed is an editorial in the *Annals of Internal Medicine* in which Susan W. Tolle (another OHSU physician) mentioned, among other things, that "the rate of admissions to hospice [in Oregon] increased 20% in 1995 and continues to increase."[93]

On the other hand, not even all those in Oregon who support the idea that doctors and patients should be free mutually to decide what is appropriate in end-of-life care have always been comfortable with the way things have worked out. An Oregon physician who helped found the Center for Ethics in Health Care at OHSU, even while echoing Quill's observations about the positive effects of the assisted-suicide law in Oregon, insisted that such a law should not be necessary. He seemed to be implying that doctors and patients should be left to settle things between themselves—as traditionally they had done.[94] But two days earlier, yet another Oregon physician, the national director of Physicians for Compassionate Care, wrote angrily and sadly that the "same organization that funds assisted suicide for the poor has restricted pain care funding for the poor. . . . In fact, in the past two years, Oregon has already begun to fall in its ranking among other states in its per-capita use of pain medications. Prescription of legitimate pain medicine for the seriously ill is being undermined by the only state that pays for assisted suicide."[95] A sober analysis of the situation by bioethics instructor Joan Woolfrey includes the caution that, at the very least, complying with the new law will put increased demands on a physician's time.[96]

Clearly, more data are needed before the whole picture is in focus. And one complicating factor is the series of efforts made by officers of the federal government in 2001 to block—indeed, to undermine—Oregon's landmark law. In early November of that year, Attorney General John D. Ashcroft, reversing an administrative decision by his predecessor (Janet Reno), sent a memorandum to the chief of the Drug Enforcement Administration "authorizing federal drug agents to identify and punish doctors who prescribe federally controlled drugs to help terminally ill patients commit suicide."[97] This is not the first effort that has been made on a federal level to interfere with the Oregon statute; it will probably not be the last.[98]

Quite independent of ODDA, incidentally, another Oregon innovation—the one-page Physician Orders for Life-Sustaining Treatment (POLST)—has played a different but also important role in improved end-of-life care in that state. Patients who do not want physician assistance in dying but

who also do not want physicians to burden them with excessive technological interventions in the dying process can, it would appear, pretty well
count on having their wishes taken seriously—at least at the OHSU
hospital. When an elderly patient with a valid POLST was intubated and
given "all the usual array of life-support," her case was seen as the "serious medical error" that those struggling against death by technology believe it to be. Steps were taken to make sure all concerned understood this
and that it would not happen again.[99]

The other legal story of significance in the United States unfolded more
or less in tandem with the debate in Oregon. In January 1997, the
U.S. Supreme Court heard arguments on two assisted-suicide cases—
Washington v. Glucksberg (out of the Ninth Circuit) and *Vacco v. Quill* (out
of the Second Circuit). The most striking fact about these two cases was
that although both arose out of decisions that struck down laws prohibiting assisted suicide (one in the state of Washington, the other in New
York), they did so for different reasons. Both courts based their rulings on
provisions of the Fourteenth Amendment. The Ninth Circuit court concluded that prohibiting assistance in dying violated the due process clause,
however, while the Second Circuit court relied on its decision on the equal
protection clause. (An elegant analysis of these Circuit court decisions,
written by Ronald Dworkin, includes among its many helpful features
Dworkin's clear and concise statement of the differences between the two
constitutional clauses. "The due process clause," he wrote, "forbids com-
promising certain basic rights altogether, except for a particularly com-
pelling reason. . . . The equal protection clause is less stringent; it requires
only that states not discriminate unfairly in the liberties and other privileges it chooses to allow."[100])

Much has been written about these cases, some of it in the form of briefs,
of course, and more of it in analysis after the fact.[101] For our purposes,
what really matters is the outcome that was announced in June 1997:
"Court, 9-0, Upholds State Laws Prohibiting Assisted Suicide," the *New
York Times* announced in a large all-caps headline. The subhead was even
more blunt: "No Help For Dying."[102] The Court did not slam the door
tightly shut, however. By upholding the existing state laws (that is, over-
turning the lower courts), the Supreme Court in its unanimous vote declared unequivocally that this was a matter for the individual states to
decide. In many ways, it was—as Timothy Quill noted—a "wise decision,
a decision where everybody won" (at least something).[103] First, the Court
did not retreat from earlier decisions affirming legal rights of patients.
And, in *Glucksberg*, the Court explicitly stated that the "holding permits
this debate to continue, as it should in a democratic society."[104]

Meanwhile, knowledge (however fragmentary) about euthanasia in
Holland has helped shape the debate in the United States. Yet some of that
shaping has been quite misleading. We need to clarify what the main

issues are and where the primary disagreements lie, and to identify the best sources for those who seek further understanding. The point is to show why what happens in Holland is not directly relevant to the issue of whether physician-assisted suicide, euthanasia, or any other form of physician-aid-in-dying should be legalized in the United States.

Until April 2001, neither "euthanasia" as we typically understand it nor "physician-assisted suicide" (as that term is generally used in the United States, also indicating a positive act on the part of the physician) was legal in Holland. In that month, the Dutch Senate (by a vote of 46–28) endorsed the Parliament of the Netherlands' lower house vote (which had passed 104–40 in November 2000) legalizing mercy killings and assisted suicide. (The law did not in fact go into effect until one year later.)[105] Prior to that, euthanasia and assisting in a suicide were both "explicitly and apparently absolutely prohibited" by the Dutch Criminal Code (articles 293 and 294).[106] What has long confused many outside Holland is that reports about euthanasia being carried out there were not necessarily accompanied by reports of physicians being prosecuted; the resulting temptation to assume that such actions must be legal is understandable, but to draw such a conclusion is to ignore the facts. In fact, those engaging in euthanasia often were prosecuted—not for helping a patient die, but rather (for instance) for failing to follow procedures or to report their actions in appropriate fashion. Sentences were generally suspended.[107] Evolving case law since the early 1970s has provided two possible defenses for euthanasia: the justification of "necessity" and the requirements of "careful practice." If doctors followed a carefully prescribed set of rules in connection with ending a patient's life and—most especially—adhered to the prescribed reporting procedures, they would not be prosecuted. The simplest way to describe in lay terms the situation before the passage of the new law is to say not that euthanasia was legal (which it was not) but that it was not (exactly) illegal.

Among the most sensible and helpful of popular press reports on the situation in Holland was a three-part series written by columnist Ellen Goodman shortly before the Supreme Court handed down its decision in *Glucksberg* and *Quill;* the trio of articles appeared in the *Boston Globe* in April 1997.[108] For Goodman, the issue arose because "somewhere along the way the right-to-die movement went from asking about stopping treatment to asking for a doctor's help in dying. Now this is at the heart of the assisted-suicide case[s] before the US Supreme Court." But even if she is right, her conviction that hints about how the debate will unfold can be found in Holland seem to me based on at least one important error: She says that in Holland, as here, the debate began "as a patients' rights movement."[109] The authors of *Euthanasia & Law in the Netherlands* directly contradict this. First, the three of them—John Griffiths, Alex Bood, and Heleen Weyers—point out that the Dutch do not make an issue of a legal distinction between euthanasia and physician-assisted suicide the way others typically do: "[O]ne of the most characteristic features of euthanasia practice in the Netherlands is that from the beginning of the public discussion until very recently there has been no suggestion of a legal preference for assistance with suicide over euthanasia in the narrow sense of killing on request. . . . [In fact,] killing on request is much more common than assistance with suicide." This preference, they go on to say, is a reflection of the development of Dutch euthanasia law, which contrasts with the situation in the United States. In the Netherlands there was less a demand for patients' rights and more an "insistence by doctors . . . that under limited circumstances euthanasia is a legitimate medical procedure."[110] The change in the law in 2001 does not undermine the accuracy of that statement.

This difference in the root of the debate has many ramifications; not least of them is the opening it provides for emphasis in the Netherlands to be laid on what counts as "requirements of careful practice." Similarly, according to the report of the Remmelink Commission,[111] "'help in dying' [is regarded] as 'normal medical practice'. . . . It seems likely that 'help in dying' has long been rather standard medical practice."[112] Though there are doctors in the United States who also argue that "help in dying" is a critical part of the continuum of care that physicians should offer their patients, there has never been an open acknowledgment of it as anything close to "normal" or "standard" medical practice. Thus this difference in the origins of the euthanasia discussion in the two countries is fundamental, and Goodman's (or anyone else's) attempt to equate the two situations is distorting. A helpful comparison can be made only if the situations in the two countries are truly comparable, and in this important regard they are not.

Another indication that Goodman has perhaps not fully grasped all the idiosyncratic nuances of the Dutch situation comes in her attempt to explain the Dutch attitude toward euthanasia by calling on the concept known in Dutch as *gedogen*. She acknowledges in her column that her informant, Gerrit van der Wal, has trouble translating it for her; she resorts (whether with van der Wal's acquiescence is unclear) to saying that *gedogen* "describes a formal condition somewhere between forbidden and permitted. It is part of the Dutch dance of principle and pragmatism."[113] But elsewhere, one of the most thoughtful and well-respected commentators on "the Dutch way," Margaret Pabst Battin, was criticized on precisely this point: "[S]he wrongly describes Dutch euthanasia law as falling under the concept of *gedogen*, or systematic toleration of violations of the law."[114] If she was wrong, so was Goodman. The difficulties with this single word are instructive, reminding us that—both literally and figuratively—something is almost always lost in the translation.

Unfortunately, many of the short editorials, newspaper reports, or op-ed columns about euthanasia in the Netherlands that have been published in the United States blur other significant details as well. Even in the more discursive analyses in professional journals, this very complicated subject has all too often been treated simplistically. Many of the books that purport to inform us how the Dutch deal with euthanasia and physician-assisted dying are also severely flawed.

Part of the difficulty remains in the fact that (especially now that the legal landscape has been modified) Holland continues to be an inappropriate model for the United States. The attempt to use the Dutch experience to make political points (less commonly ethical or medical ones) both distorts the actual Dutch situation and tells us little about our own. Griffiths, Bood, and Weyers agree: "On the whole, the descriptions of Dutch law and practice concerning euthanasia available in English are either so uncritically apologetic, or so obviously and even maliciously biassed, that the reader who is looking not for an advocate's brief or an exercise in axe-grinding but just a straightforward presentation of the evidence is left not knowing what to believe."[115]

These authors are willing to praise good work. Though they took issue with Battin's understanding of *gedogen,* they also characterized her as a "lonely exception" to the general rule quoted just above. Her "account of the Dutch situation," they say, "is, as far as the essentials are concerned, objective and critical."[116] They go on to say that Carlos Gomez and John Keown are "the most responsible exponents" of the position that accepts "in principle many of the supporting arguments in favor of Dutch euthanasia practice" but then rejects it on the ground that it "is not, and cannot be, adequately controlled"[117]—before they proceed forcefully to show where Gomez and Keown go wrong. While Keown "is reasonably accurate with regard to Dutch law and respectful of empirical data," his argument "is actually a boomerang."[118] And far worse, according to these authors, Gomez relies on information gathered in a manner that "can only be described as scientifically irresponsible."[119]

My own view of Gomez's major work on the subject, *Regulating Death: Euthanasia and the Case of the Netherlands* (1991), is fully consonant with this assessment. Though he was far more balanced and moderate than Herbert Hendin (about whom more will follow), he also stumbled into trouble, among other things by placing enormous weight on his own interpretation of the way certain professional jargon is used in Dutch.[120] On the strength of what he makes his claim that the Dutch are engaged in "an active sort of deception" is unclear; neither does he have sufficient glue to make his pronouncements stick when he observes that "a liberal democracy limits what the state may and may not regulate" and that "the situation in Holland is not so benign."[121]

The most vigorous criticism is reserved by Griffiths and his colleagues for Herbert Hendin, quite appropriately. Hendin's attacks on the Dutch approach to euthanasia have appeared in many places. In a *New York Times* op-ed piece, he bombarded his readers with his extremist views without giving any indication of the basis for his claims. He asserted, for example, that his "four years of research on assisted suicide and euthanasia . . . show that Dutch doctors . . . invariably support the relatives' desire to be free of the burden of caring for the patient," and that his work "also shows that acceptance of euthanasia in the Netherlands has reduced interest in alleviating pain and suffering; euthanasia becomes an easier alternative."[122] In addition to writing various articles, Hendin turned one of them into a book, *Seduced by Death: Doctors, Patients and the Dutch Cure* (1997). The salient feature of this all-out attack on the Dutch way of handling euthanasia is the strident and self-confident (not to say smug and self-satisfied) tone of the author. Insisting that he began with an open mind, Hendin gives every sign of not having done so and of having fallen into precisely the pattern he criticizes in others: "Physicians and the public often come to the question of euthanasia with their minds made up."[123] He condescends: Timothy Quill and Herbert Cohen (a leading Dutch doctor in the field of euthanasia; see my Profile of him that follows) are, he acknowledges, "compassionate and concerned physicians," but they let their suicidal patients use them. He is sarcastic: "[M]ost people understand and accept the distinction between killing and allowing to die" (implying "what's wrong with these people that they don't?"). He makes vague and sweeping judgments: "[E]uthanasia brings out the worst" in medicine.[124] Most telling is the way Hendin explains—always negatively— everything the supporters of physician-aid-in-dying say and then lets the views of those opposed to euthanasia stand without interpretation, as if their words expressed self-evident truths. In sum, as Griffiths, Bood, and Weyers say in *Euthanasia & Law,* Hendin's "'findings which supposedly support his conclusions are so filled with mistakes of law, of fact, and of interpretation, mostly tendentious, that it is hard to be charitable and regard them as merely negligent." He is, they add one page later, "also breathtakingly arrogant."[125]

Do any features of the situation in Holland tell us what legalizing physician-aid-in-dying in the United States might be like? It is clear that the issue of the number and frequency of euthanasia cases without an explicit patient request concerns the Dutch every bit as much as it does thoughtful persons anywhere (this is also independent of the recent change in the law). In a book of essays reporting research on the overall euthanasia and assisted-suicide debate in the Netherlands, Gerrit van der Wal uses the publication of the "Debbie" story to introduce precisely this topic.[126] But as Derek Humphry pointed out in a letter to the *JAMA* editor, the story in fact tells us nothing about Holland; any Dutch physician who acted in this manner would have been subject to prosecution.[127] (Again, the Dutch law that went into effect in April 2002 does not make this any less true today.) Pointing out that prior to the work of the Remmelink Commission, there were few data available on the subject in Holland, he proceeds to explain his own research. One of van der Wal's summarizing comments near the end of his meticulous report is that, in general, "euthanasia and assisted suicide are nowhere nearly so frequent as has for a long time been thought, especially outside Holland." That notwithstanding, he also cautions two pages later that "it is altogether possible that the quality of the medical and technical performance of euthanasia can be improved."[128]

Importantly—but apparently not widely known in the United States— van der Wal's total of euthanasia cases without explicit request from the patient was roughly 100 a year in the practice of family doctors. The number of non-voluntary euthanasia cases (that is, cases where there was no specific request from the patient—*not* instances of *in*voluntary euthanasia, carried out *against* the patient's wishes) that the Remmelink Commission claimed to have found was 1,000 per year. Granted, there are some differences in the research methods used by van der Wal and Remmelink. Still, it seems highly likely that the majority of the cases Remmelink reported were found in hospitals (and to a lesser extent in nursing homes) rather than in the private practices of family physicians. Van der Wal's much lower figure is significant because most of the worries about regulation in Holland have had to do with the difficulty of knowing what family physicians do in the privacy of their offices or their patients' homes. Unlike their counterparts in the United States, they see the majority of their patients in these settings (and thus far from prying eyes or any easily set-up system of monitoring).[129] Second, attention has not been paid in the United States to the near impossibility of making trustworthy estimates (a matter much discussed in the Dutch literature), given how the original interview questions were posed.[130] Further confusing the issue of the exact numbers is that a later replication of the Remmelink study concluded the number was 900 instead of 1,000.[131] Despite the importance of acknowledging that cases of non-voluntary euthanasia may be taking place in the Netherlands (and elsewhere, for that matter), reducing the discussion to one of quibbling over the precise numbers helps no one.

A dramatic example of how the Dutch data have been distorted can be found in the work of even a sophisticated and thoughtful writer like Daniel Callahan. In Holland, he has shrilly insisted, there is "widespread abuse (at least 1,000 patients a year put to death without their permission) and a general flouting of the law. There is no reason the same thing would not happen here."[132] In his eagerness to press the argument against the legalization of euthanasia, Callahan appears to have accepted the figure of 1,000 completely uncritically and then to have drawn dire conclusions about what legalization in the United States would mean. He made no effort to explain the circumstances of these deaths or the difficulties Dutch researchers themselves have found in clarifying precisely what the figure represents. Nor did he make an effort to explain that these deaths were in any case instances of non-voluntary euthanasia, not to be confused with involuntary euthanasia. Callahan relies on rhetorical tricks, using loaded phrases ("widespread abuse," "general flouting of the law") and making unsubstantiated claims ("there is no reason the same thing would not happen here") instead of acknowledging that what is at issue is basically an empirical question. The result is that it becomes both easy and necessary simply to dismiss his argument as irrelevant.

Moreover, the central matter ought to be not so much the details of what goes on in the Netherlands as whether—whatever *does* go on there—it is an appropriate model for the United States. Is "the Dutch way" exportable, in other words? The answer must be negative. This does not mean there is no value in seeking to understand how the Dutch handle this sensitive political, legal, medical, ethical, and personal subject; any insight on such a difficult topic is bound to be helpful. But to draw conclusions from such an analysis about what the outcome of a similar approach would be in the United States is to fail to take adequately into account the enormous differences between the social setting and history in Holland, for instance, and our own social circumstances and history. For one thing, not even 1 percent of the Dutch population is without health insurance.[133] Doctors in Holland, like those in England, gain nothing financially either by under-treating or by over-treating their patients; there is no danger that financial considerations will influence the treatment of particularly vulnerable patients facing the end of life.

The best work showing why Holland is not an appropriate model for the United States has been done by Margaret Pabst Battin.[134] Among the "dozen caveats" she offers, perhaps the central ones are those that point to cultural differences. She details some of the factors that cannot easily be altered or wished away: "The institutional circumstances of euthanasia in the Netherlands are easily misunderstood," "Terminological differences operate to confuse the issue," "The Dutch see the role of law rather differently," "The economic circumstances of euthanasia in the Netherlands are also easily misunderstood."[135]

On the other hand, Battin is uncomfortable concluding we can never "be like the Dutch" if such a conclusion means ruling out the possibility of euthanasia, because the desirability of having physician-aid-in-dying available is so manifest to her. "My own view," she writes, "is that it is a matter of fundamental right for the person facing an intolerable end to expect help from his or her physician in the matter of dying." For the nonce, she grants that we may have to live with a compromise—another way of saying that, at least for the time being, each of us will have to lay his or her own corduroy road through the wilderness and the swamp.[136] Since Dutch socio-political customs are what drive "the Dutch way" in this particular arena of medical care (as well as in others), and since those customs are not the same as ours, we can hardly expect "the Dutch way" to fit, here. We must find our own way.

PROFILE: HERBERT COHEN[137]

The amount of time I have available for an interview during my stay in Holland is not great. Although the prospect of an excuse to visit Rotterdam and its environs to interview Dr. Herbert Cohen is welcome, it is not clear that a side trip there is actually feasible. So I am relieved when Cohen sweeps the problem away not only by responding affirmatively to my request for an interview but also by volunteering to undertake the journey to Amsterdam. He is always happy for an excuse to visit Amsterdam, he tells me, managing in the process to make it sound as if I have done him a favor by asking for some of his time.

And time he gives me. He meets me in the lobby of my hotel precisely as arranged, and I am immediately charmed by his open and friendly manner, his cheerful smile, his eagerness to accommodate. Cohen is a splendid prototype of one type of Dutchman—not very tall, maybe a little over-weight, a broad and handsome face. I can imagine him, in an earlier period, sitting for Frans Hals. The portrait would have had to be like Hals's famous "Laughing Cavalier" that is part of the Wallace Collection in London, however. I see nothing in the man before me of the self-important poses of the civic guards so typical of Hals's group-portrait paintings.

We talk before lunch and on the way to a nearby restaurant; we talk steadily through lunch and for another couple of hours after lunch, throughout a meandering walk in Vondel Park. (Cohen tells me I have to see the place, that it is the perfect illustration of Amsterdam's anything-goes policies. He presses this mini-excursion on me with cheerful urgency, proud of his country's tolerant attitude toward all.)

Quickly it becomes clear that Cohen has had considerable experience explaining Holland's unique approach to physician-assisted suicide and euthanasia, but he shows no signs of being bored by the request to do it again. Nor is the need to explain it all in English any barrier; like so many of his fellow citizens, he speaks English with an ease and fluency fully consonant with his mastery of the subject at hand. His vigorous manner and lively account of his ongoing involvement in euthanasia utterly belie the picture Herbert Hendin painted of him as a weary old doctor who had to give up his medical practice, plagued by lingering doubts he would not or could not admit.[138] I find instead that I am in the company of a man who expresses himself firmly but thoughtfully; he is content, not smug.

Indeed, although he cannot resist reporting that he was recently named to the Queen's Honors List, he seems genuinely ambivalent over what the most appropriate response to the honor should be. He is torn between being slightly amused and truly pleased. "I am conservative [in the practice of euthanasia]; that's why the government likes me," he says with a mischievous grin. More seriously, he stresses that the importance of his having been thus honored is that it constitutes very public support for the special kind of contribution to people's welfare he truly believes the practice of euthanasia can make.

Cohen gives every evidence of carrying his years of experience well. Among other things, he takes very seriously his position as the oldest (in terms of service) of those who have performed euthanasia, which brings with it some responsibilities. One of those implicit responsibilities is talking with people like me. Another, more important, is teaching a course for the Dutch Medical Association aimed at improving the quality of the practice of euthanasia; the course is taught jointly with a palliative-care expert. He also teaches (at three universities) special one-day sessions on euthanasia for family practitioners.

He has words of praise for some aspects of what Hospice has done—their "great work in painkilling and in the use of morphine," for example. But he is disdainful of the Hospice line that performing euthanasia will erode trust between doctors and patients. "If you shout that from the rooftops loud enough, it will seem to be true," he mutters. He obviously doesn't believe it at all, stressing that the task of working out whether euthanasia is the best option for a given patient can take a lot of time—up to three years of visits and discussion and exploration of other options. And although in a technical sense it is "chillingly easy" to perform euthanasia, it is also a "horrible" and weighty experience. "The only thing more horrible is the second time, because you remember the first time." (I am struck at how the emotional earnestness with which he makes the comment is once again in complete contrast to a claim made by Herbert Hendin, namely that a "quite troubling thing happens to the physicians who participate in this. . . . The first assisted suicide may give them a moment's pause. The second is easier. It eventually turns into a kind of compulsion."[139]) Cohen insists that even when everything possible has been done to make sure the patient is ready, when the patient has been reminded it is possible to back down, when the doctor has re-iterated a willingness "to go home and come back when you call"—it is still very difficult. A doctor's "skill is not at its best at such a moment." Euthanasia is not an easy way out, for doctors or for patients—who, Cohen tells me, really have to fight for euthanasia.

Cohen's qualities as a teacher emerge vividly when he reaches for a piece of paper (eventually it takes several) so he can sketch for me the complicated route that a doctor who performs euthanasia in Holland must follow. What becomes absolutely clear is that no doctor who adheres to the prescribed procedure is engaged in a simple means of dealing with a dying patient. The contrast with Kevorkian's modus operandi could not be more pronounced. As for whether euthanasia not being legal might mean that some doctors prefer not to bother with all the proper procedures (not wanting to be on record as having performed euthanasia), Cohen concedes legalization might make it easier for some physicians to follow through. But he has been said to be "in no hurry to see euthanasia legalised," believing the difficulties of interpretation in any Act could raise more problems than they would solve.[140]

This coincides with what he said publicly at the 10th International Conference of the World Federation of Right to Die Societies in Bath, England (in 1994). Fighting for legislation on euthanasia should not be the primary goal because there are "social preconditions" that need to be in place. First, there has to be access to adequate health-care services (especially palliative care); then there has to be an educated public, a general attitude of tolerance across society, "mature" doctor-patient relationships, and the availability to all of family physicians.[141]

Just as Cohen believes euthanasia is not solely a matter for the law, he does not think it should be a wholly medical matter. "I like the spiritual to play a role," he says. And when he does perform euthanasia, he likes to get the essential medical equipment in place ahead of time, in order to avoid turning the solemn event, carrying out euthanasia, into a strictly medical occasion. It should be a ceremony, *"een liturgie,"* he tells me, lapsing into Dutch for the first and only time during our conversation. Cohen's conviction that the moment of a chosen death is one of profundity is palpable.

I suspect he has views on everyone and everything connected with death and dying, though of course we do not have time to explore them all. He does tell me that Elisabeth Kübler-Ross made "the greatest breakthrough." That Margaret Pabst Battin is right—the Dutch form of euthanasia is absolutely not exportable (and the reasons she gives are correct). That John Griffiths and his co-authors are too taken with the idea that "the walls are porous" between euthanasia and assisted suicide (Cohen thinks the compartments are more sharply divided from each other, and that assisted suicide is even more difficult for the doctor because the outcome is less certain). As for Bert Keizer (whose book *Dancing With Mr. D* I mentioned earlier[142]), he is "a wise clown." Cohen smiles and chuckles. "All the nice people have a streak of madness in them," he laughs. And so I do not learn what Cohen really thinks of either the book or doctor-author Keizer with his zany and offbeat way of presenting serious stories about deaths he has attended.

Would I want Dr. Herbert Cohen to be my attending physician near the end of life? After hours in his company, listening to his earnest discussion of how and why death—for some patients—is best achieved by a doctor performing euthanasia, I would unhesitatingly say "yes." Cohen has enlivened the middle of this day spent talking about death and dying. One sentence in particular echoes in my head after we part company: "What counts with me is the biography of the patient," Cohen says. In other words, patients' *lives* are what matter most to him as he helps them with their deaths.

MEDICAL HELP

One of the chief factors in the shifting shape of both public and private discourse on matters having to do with death and dying are fundamental changes (or perceived changes), during recent years, in the way doctors and patients relate to each other. Two features of the medical world in the United States today that loom especially large have profound implications for the doctor-patient relationship: the increased use of medical technology and the growing dominance of health maintenance organizations (HMOs). Some of the concerns raised by the stories of Janet Adkins and "Debbie" are directly traceable to these now-characteristic elements of how modern medicine is practiced. The "do-it-yourself help" that Kevorkian represents, with its reliance on gadgetry, looks like an extreme but understandable development of what can happen in a medical world where technology sometimes comes between doctor and patient. The help that might be available if physician-aid-in-dying were legalized looks equally (though differently) unattractive to many; the likelihood of frequent middle-of-the-night endings of lives at the solitary discretion of a doctor, with no personal relationship between doctor and patient required, appears too great. If these two kinds of options are undesirable or unavailable, where does that leave us? Do we have any other options? We need to explore whether within the confines of the modern doctor-patient relationship there is enough flexibility and room for medical help with the actual dying process, with or without legalization.

It is tempting to grow sentimental over the "good old days" of medicine, a supposedly simpler age when the family doctor was a fixture on the local scene and knew his patients through their entire lives. This romantic view can be only partially supported by historical facts. For one thing, by no means everyone had access to care, and some of the doctors were no doubt ill trained if not downright incompetent. Furthermore, a great deal of what we now take for granted as basic medicine was not known until relatively recent times. In addition, leaving aside the negatives, there is at least one positive reason for not waxing nostalgic. The best of what doctors from this putative Golden Age of Medicine offered is still available, in principle, today: a thoughtful and caring concern for

patients and a willingness to spend time with them through difficult, painful, and even life-ending episodes of illness and disease.

As Daniel Callahan has pointed out (sounding considerably less
partisan than when he discusses euthanasia), "Caring should always take
priority over curing for the most obvious of reasons: There is never any
certainty that our illnesses can be cured or our death averted. Eventually
they will, and must, triumph. Our victories over sickness and death are
always temporary, but our need for support, for caring . . . is always permanent." Nor is it mindlessly old fashioned to urge the priority of caring
over curing. "The steady increase in chronic illness, the almost certain
emergence of economic limits on many curative possibilities, and dis-
satisfaction with impersonal medicine press it once again to the fore-
ground."[143] Part of what makes Callahan's analysis helpful is his
clear-eyed insistence on not letting technological imperatives (what he
calls "technological brinkmanship") take over.[144]

The great danger in technological boom-times is that doctors will become enamored of all the elaborate things they *can* do and lose sight of
the basic questions: Who is in charge? Whose life (or death) is it, anyway?
The world where it was deemed appropriate for patients to "follow
doctor's orders" unquestioningly is forever behind us. While it certainly
makes sense under many circumstances to take advantage of the improvements in care and diagnosis that technology (loosely and broadly defined)
offers, it is also true that there is no substitute for doctors and patients
actually talking to each other.[145] Furthermore, although Callahan's observations on this point are insightful, his apparently settled views on euthanasia and other forms of physician-aid-in-dying tend to stifle debate.
In a thoughtful discussion on the subject in his *What Kind of Life?* (1990),
he states more than once that "the most potent motive at present for active
euthanasia and assisted suicide is that of a dread of the power of medicine."[146] Unfortunately, he stops there, seemingly unwilling to acknowledge that helping someone die might itself be a manifestation of precisely
the kind of "caring" he touts all along. What Timothy Quill sees as a logical
continuum of care (see my Profile of him that follows), Daniel Callahan
sees only in terms of a doctor's loss of his moral compass. Callahan also
argues adamantly in favor of maintaining a distinction between "killing"
and "letting die." But as I endeavored to show in Chapter 3, that distinction is not likely to settle the central issues (certainly not in every instance)
when it comes to making medical decisions at the end of life.

The key to how such questions were traditionally answered was the
doctor's accepted position of authority. Thus physicians could—and many
of them did—"ease the passage" (from life to death) of untold numbers
of patients.[147] The modern move away from an authoritarian model of the
good doctor means that we cannot and no longer do assume the doctor

always knows and does what is best. As patients, we want to take an active part in our own medical lives at least some of the time, perhaps especially when it comes to end-of-life matters.

Where does this leave us, given the high-tech, HMO-dominated world in which we live? The first step, surely, is to recall that one main responsibility of physicians is to respond to patients' desires to have their suffering relieved. Not that we do not know this—and also not that we are unaware how crucial the development of a good relationship between doctors and patients is. But we still seem to need reminding that, as one physician pointed out, there "can be a workable relationship between patient and doctor that takes into account the patient's feelings and intelligence while still recognizing the doctor's specialized knowledge and informed judgment."[148] The headline over the *New York Times* report of a later study trumpeted what should not have been a surprise: "Doctors Find Comfort Is a Potent Medicine."[149] But another more recent headline in the same paper tells a different story: "Doctors Say H.M.O.'s Limit What They Can Tell Patients."[150] Bob Herbert, likewise writing in the *New York Times* (another year after that), quoted doctors who were worried that HMOs and all they represent were "destroying the doctor-patient relationship."[151]

What we may need is a new-old view of what lifelong assistance from our physicians should mean. We have no trouble with the idea of asking physicians to help during the very natural process of a baby being born; perhaps we need to cultivate some parallel thinking about the very natural process of dying. This is what makes so evocative the idea of a doctor being "a midwife through the dying process" (an expression I used earlier and that Timothy Quill uses as a book title). Why should doctors not assist us in leaving the world as well as in entering it?

Some people clearly think that assistance with dying is indeed the ultimate gift of the caring physician. Patients cry out for such help: "I searched long and hard to find a doctor . . . to honor my ability to make my own medical decisions," writes one. "I am a cancer patient. It would give me great comfort to know that if I were suffering unendurable pain . . .—with the help of a trusted physician—I could end my life without losing dignity and without enduring prolonged suffering," writes another.[152] Doctors, too, have gone public in print, in some cases arguing in favor of legalizing physician-assisted suicide: "In the very few cases where suicide is appropriate and the circumstances are well documented and regulated, doctors should be able to give assistance. Just as important, the patients who fear unrelievable suffering at the end of life need creditable assurance that assistance will be available should they want suicide."[153] Others, with a hopeful eye on the future, believe that doctors need to make up their minds—and preferably let their patients know—where they stand: "This matter has now reached the stage where all physicians should declare their credo, at least to themselves. It is my credo that assisting people to leave the dwelling place of their body when it is no longer habitable is becoming an obligation of the medical profession. It is part of the doctor's job," wrote a retired Harvard physician in 1995.[154] When we think about our options, we need to consider the extent to which we believe that physician-aid-in-dying should remain something between doctor and patient.

PROFILE: TIMOTHY QUILL[155]

When I mentioned to people who know Timothy Quill that I was going to Rochester to meet him, I received universally the same response: "You'll like him. He is a terrific guy." They shouldn't have said this, of course; I felt I was being set up. On the other hand, I certainly hoped they were right, because I was making a special trip to talk to him. I was in no mood for the experience to prove difficult.

I needn't have worried.

Though I am late for my appointment, getting lost in the labyrinth of hospital corridors, Dr. Quill puts me immediately at ease. When I embarrass myself by not being able to make my cassette recorder function, he also sorts that out for me. Now I can devote my full attention to what turns out to be almost an hour of relaxed but earnest conversation.

The beard and the glasses, which on some people serve as a kind of mask, instead give Timothy Quill an air of informality that perfectly matches his shirtsleeve attire. I have to suppress a smile as I recall the way one newspaper article about him began: "More Marcus Welby than Jack Kevorkian."[156] Absolutely. He appears comfortable with himself, which no doubt is part of what enables him to be such an accommodating person and makes it easy for people to like and trust him.

Before my visit, I had read two of Quill's books; I now quickly ascertain that his writing forms a seamless whole with what emerges when he speaks. I hear almost nothing that surprises me as this quiet, thoughtful doctor answers my questions; he is a superb listener, as well. What he believes, what he does, and what he urges on others all fit together. The depth and breadth of his experience, and the thoughtfulness of his reflections on the subject of caring for terminally ill patients, are undeniable. No wonder he is referred to as "a leading voice in the controversy over physician-assisted death"—as the jacket copy of his book *A Midwife Through the Dying Process* (1996) has it.[157] Or, as law professor Laurence H. Tribe (who argued *Vacco v. Quill* before the Supreme Court in January 1997) is quoted as saying, he is "a good representative of what *ought* to happen, because death is not his subspecialty but an integrated part of his practice."[158]

Although Quill's books are full of stories about individual patients, the decisions he (and they) faced, and the lessons learned, our wide-ranging conversation is mostly more philosophical and general. Clearly Timothy Quill is more than a storyteller. Only twice does he mention particular cases to me. Once, explaining his reaction to a critic, he talks (again) about his patient Diane, whose case he had written up in the *NEJM*. And in recounting his experience at St. Christopher's Hospice outside of London, he mentions one of the patients he saw there to make a point about what he thinks is wrong with the most rigid and doctrinaire aspects of the Hospice ideology. Otherwise, we talk issues.

The single most important message I receive in talking with Quill is his utter and absolute certainty that "Hospice . . . is the standard of care, for people who are dying, against which everything else should be measured." To be sure, Timothy Quill is a proponent of physician-assisted death where it is called for; he is someone "at the frontier of social change," as has been said.[159] Though there is no question that he came to prominence as a result of publishing the story of how he helped Diane make her suicide "possible, successful, and relatively painless,"[160] there is far more to his career than that. He has himself been medical director of a Hospice unit, and he continues to press vigorously for Hospice-type care. "I believe very strongly in Hospice," he tells me; "I never talk about assisted dying without talking about hospice care." To do otherwise, he stresses, makes no sense. Listening to him, I find it hard to see how anyone could say, as the writer of one letter to the editor in the *New York Times* did, that "Dr. Quill long ago dropped the cautions that once distinguished his stance from that of Dr. Jack Kevorkian's."[161] No one who knows Quill or has listened to him talk about his relationship with dying patients could possibly have made such a remark in earnest. "Caution" is Quill's middle name.

In other words, in his view, Hospice care and assisted suicide are by no means mutually exclusive. What concerns Timothy Quill, however, is that although there are many Hospice "mantras" that sound good—"Hospice care neither hastens nor prolongs dying"; "Hospice acknowledges death as a part of life"; and so on—precisely what they mean is not always so clear. He agrees with me that intoning "Hospice affirms life" is a way of taking the rhetorical high ground, as if those outside the immediate Hospice fold somehow do *not* affirm life.

Having said that, Quill is quick to point out the dangers of grouping all Hospice people (or all Hospices) together. It is "very variable" from Hospice to Hospice, he says, as to how free people feel to talk about wanting to die and how willing Hospice staff are to listen. He recounts an experience he had in Louisiana, when he visited there to speak on assisted dying. Two Hospice directors who attended the lecture spoke up. One insisted that nobody at his Hospice ever talked about wanting to die—because, he said, the staff was so successful in doing everything that was necessary for the patients to feel they were truly living until they died.

Then the second Hospice director said something to the effect of "Well, about half of our patients want to talk about it, and we let them." I am left with no doubt that Quill is much more comfortable with what transpires under the influence and leadership of that second Hospice director.

While most good Hospice directors will tolerate open discussion from patients about refusing to eat, for instance, explicit talk about wanting to die is likely to make many Hospice directors (and their staffs and the volunteers) very uncomfortable. Yet, Quill insists, these are conversations people very much need to have, at least with "the intimate others in their lives." One can see how he might become just such an "intimate other" for a patient who does not want to burden friends and family or has little support otherwise. Quill exudes a non-judgmental manner; the most private person should be comfortable talking to him.

A second point of concern for Quill is that the matter of how we die is too important—too central to the way we live at the end of our lives—to be left wholly to chance. "In other areas of medical care we do not tolerate the variations that occur around care of the dying," he says, shaking his head sadly. Clearly he thinks we should not tolerate such differences here, either. People who are dying really need to be able to have conversations about death; their caregivers, inside Hospice and outside, *must* be open to the conversation. We need protocols, and we need to train physicians so they know how and are willing to conduct such conversations.

I ask Quill what he thinks of the way so many Hospice supporters depend on the doctrine of double effect, and this time I *am* surprised by his answer. What I discover is just how tolerant he is. "I have a complicated view of the doctrine of double effect," he told me. "For people who believe in it, it is very important; it allows both patients and doctors a kind of escape route, which is useful when doctor and patient do not agree." Thanks to the doctrine, "lots of people get help who otherwise wouldn't." Patients who could never ask directly for help in dying can ask for pain relief. Likewise, doctors who would never be willing to act with direct intent to end a patient's life can comfort themselves with the knowledge that all they really wanted was to relieve the patient's pain, even if they can foresee that the amount of medication they are giving will shorten the person's life.

I argue that such double-talk is disingenuous. Quill's reply is pragmatic: If you can ease the dying process for people, he seems to be saying, it doesn't matter. It is not necessary always to get down to the deep subconscious of what it is people are "really saying and thinking; it is enough, if they get the help they need." Hmm, so the end justifies the means, I am somewhat unkindly thinking. "In a culture as diverse as ours," he responds to the question he apparently guesses is in my mind, "you have to have a lot of different approaches."

He admits, however, that when conversations are conducted under such circumstances they tend to become rather "Byzantine"—and that this is extremely unfortunate. The time one spends preparing for death "is not a time for being coy." When people start talking to each other in coded conversations, there is also always a danger they won't understand each other's codes. An open and straightforward discussion about the way one is dying is much to be preferred. What it comes down to, finally, Quill believes, is "who's in charge of the dying process." He is clear about this: It ought to be the patient. Caregivers do not need to take charge and *direct* the performance so much. Instead, they should be prepared to say to their dying patients something like "here are some options and opportunities" for you to consider as you think about how your particular story is going to end.

Quill's insistence that getting discussion out in the open is bound to improve care for the dying is engagingly stubborn. The man obviously feels strongly—and I like him for it. The real problem up to now (and still, outside Oregon) is that the whole issue of physicians' assisting in deaths has been kept underground; the deciding issue in whether patients can get assistance with death has been whether the doctor was willing to take a risk. This, Quill insists, is neither fair nor reasonable. Avoiding the risk (as much as possible) means not talking about it—but that then means both that the physician cannot consult with a colleague and that the "intimate others" in a patient's life cannot be involved. Likewise, it quite possibly means some people end up getting "assisted" with their deaths who shouldn't, and some who truly need assistance never get it.

Our conversation ends on a personal note, which puts everything Quill has said so far into a context doctors and patients alike can understand. He is suddenly talking not just as a caring physician, but as one who—like the rest of us—knows that one day he, too, will die. "You definitely want [end-of-life care] on a continuum," he says in response to one of my questions. "The worst thing is having the doctor walk away." And then: "If you can get at the notion . . . that this is your story, that my death is my story. . . ." His voice drifts off a bit, and then he continues: "I know when I am dying, I sure want a partner—a family member, of course, but also a medical partner if at all possible." This, I think to myself, is the kind of doctor I want around when I am dying: thoughtful, careful, and caring—with sound judgment on just what kind of "assistance" I might need and want when I ask for "physician assistance in dying."

NOTES

1. Denise Levertov, from "Death Psalm: O Lord of Mysteries," in *Life in the Forest* (New York: New Directions, 1978), p. 40. I am indebted to Donna Hollenberg for tracking down the poem for me.

2. The topics ranged widely. Transcripts of the entire program, "The End of Life: Exploring Death in America," can be found at *www.NPR.org* (archives, programs).

3. Jack Thomas, "A Professor's Final Course: His Own Death," *BG* (9 Mar. 1995): 55, 60.

4. Cynthia Andrews (letter to the editor), "Brandeis professor is a study in courage," *BG* (15 Mar. 1995): 14.

5. James A. Duffy, "Morris Schwartz, used own illness to teach others about living; at 78," *BG* (5 Nov. 1995): 79; [Editorial], "A teacher to the end," *BG* (13 Nov. 1995): 14; and Charles Derber (letter to the editor), "Brandeis' Schwartz would have comforted the grievers," *BG* (11 Nov. 1995): 15.

6. Mitch Albom, *Tuesdays with Morrie: An Old Man, Young Man, and Life's Greatest Lesson* (New York: Doubleday, 1997).

7. Michael Kenney, "Blunt lessons on confronting life's end," *BG* (11 Sept. 1997): E1, E7.

8. Tom Kuntz, "A Death On-Line Shows A Cyberspace With Heart and Soul," *NYT* (23 Apr. 1995): 9. The report also includes excerpts from some of the more than 2,500 responses to Mandel's announcement of his illness and subsequent updates over a five-month period.

9. Annie Calovich, "Swift end to a life of faith is shared in heartfelt e-mails," *BG* (24 Nov. 2000): A8; Ching-Ching Ni, "Dying Chinese reaches out to countrymen via Internet," *BG* (3 Dec. 2000): A24, A25.

10. Jack Kevorkian, *Prescription: Medicide* (Buffalo, N.Y.: Prometheus Books, 1991), pp. 211–31. But see also, e.g., Timothy Egan, "'Her Mind was Everything,' Dead Woman's Husband Says," *NYT* (6 June 1990): B6; David Firestone, "Doctor 'Crossed the Line,'" *Newsday* (6 June 1990): 5; "Doctor Aided Patient's Suicide," *St. Louis Post-Dispatch* (6 June 1990): 1A; and Malcolm Gladwell and William Booth, "Doctor Helps Woman Commit Suicide; Apparent Medical Assistance in Death Raises Ethical, Legal Issues," *Washington Post* (6 June 1990): A3.

11. Kevorkian, *Medicide*, p. 222. For a wholly *un*emotional argument against physician-aid-in-dying for non-terminal patients (with no reference to Jack Kevorkian), see Martin Gunderson and David J. Mayo, "Restricting Physician-Assisted Death to the Terminally Ill," *HCR* 30, no. 6 (Nov./Dec. 2000): 17–23.

12. Isabel Wilkerson, "Talk of Suicide and a Search for Death," *NYT* (9 Jan. 1991): A14.

13. Anonymous, "It's Over, Debbie," *JAMA* 259, no. 2 (8 Jan. 1988): 272. A later editorial reported that reactions "from the public and media were delayed but were extraordinary in volume and duration." George Lundberg, "'It's Over, Debbie' and the Euthanasia Debate," *JAMA* 259, no. 14 (8 Apr. 1988): 2142.

14. Willard Gaylin, Leon R. Kass, Edmund D. Pellegrino, and Mark Siegler, "Doctors Must Not Kill," *JAMA* 259, no. 14 (8 Apr. 1988): 2139, 2140.

15. Kenneth L. Vaux, "Debbie's Dying: Mercy Killing and the Good Death," *JAMA* 259, no. 14 (8 Apr. 1988): 2140, 2141.

16. See (letters to the editor), "It's Over, Debbie," *JAMA* 259, no. 14 (8 Apr. 1988): 2094–98.

17. Lundberg, "'It's Over, Debbie,'" *JAMA*: 2142, 2143.

18. Timothy E. Quill, "Death and Dignity: A Case of Individualized Decision Making," *NEJM* 324, no. 10 (7 Mar. 1991): 691–94.

19. Quill, "Death and Dignity," *NEJM*: 693.

20. Quill, "Death and Dignity," *NEJM*: 694.

21. Quill, "Death and Dignity," *NEJM*: 694 (emphasis added).

22. Quill, "Death and Dignity," *NEJM*: 694.

23. Timothy E. Quill, *Death and Dignity: Making Choices and Taking Charge* (New York: Norton, 1993), p. 17.

24. Quill, *Death and Dignity*, p. 23.

25. Quill, *Death and Dignity*, p. 17.

26. Mark A. Brunelli, "West Roxbury man is latest apparent Kevorkian suicide," *BG* (7 Mar. 1998): B3.

27. See, e.g., Larry Tye, "Focus shifts in assisted-suicide debate," *BG* (9 Feb. 1998): A1; and [Editorial], "New Kevorkian direction is feared," *BG* (2 Mar. 1998): A5.

28. Raja Mishra, "A study of deaths raises questions on Kevorkian image," *BG* (7 Dec. 2000): A3.

29. On a PBS "Frontline" program shown on Boston's Channel 2 on 14 May 1996, "The Kevorkian Verdict," bio-ethicist Arthur Caplan said Jack Kevorkian would probably be remembered as the "central figure who made Americans grapple with the question of assisted suicide."

30. Lonny Shavelson, *A Chosen Death: The Dying Confront Assisted Suicide* (Berkeley: University of California Press, 1998 [New York: Simon & Schuster, 1995]), pp. 68–104.

31. An exception appeared late in 1998, though the "crime" was considerably less remarkable. See "In first conviction, Kevorkian found guilty of assault, resisting arrest," *BG* (5 Nov. 1998): A31. Even after a videotape provided by Kevorkian that showed him actually injecting a patient with lethal drugs was shown on national television (discussion of this will follow), speculation was rife that a jury might still be unwilling to convict Kevorkian of murder; see Pam Belluck, "For Kevorkian, a Fifth, but Very Different, Trial," *NYT* (20 Mar. 1999): A1, A10. In the event, he was convicted (of second-degree murder). Dirk Johnson, "Kevorkian Sentenced to 10 to 25 Years in Prison," *NYT* (14 Apr. 1999): A1, A21.

32. Timothy E. Quill and Betty Rollin, "Dr. Kevorkian Runs Wild," *NYT* (29 Aug. 1996): A25.

33. Derek Humphry and Mary Clement, *Freedom to Die: People, Politics, and the Right-to-Die Movement* (New York: St. Martin's, 1998), pp. 126, 127, 142.

34. Timothy Quill, personal communication.

35. Quill and Rollin, "Dr. Kevorkian Runs Wild," *NYT*: A25.

36. Jack Lessenberry, "The journey of Dr. Kevorkian," *BG* (4 June 1995): 8.

37. "Kevorkian wins foundation award," *BG* (1 Dec. 1995): 13.

38. "Doctors Offer Some Support To Kevorkian," *NYT* (5 Dec. 1995): A21.

39. "Kevorkian lauded by British journal," *BG* (9 June 1996): 11.

40. Frank A. Oski, "Opting Out," *The Nation* 258, no. 3 (24 Jan. 1994): 77.

41. Greg Pence, "Dr. Kevorkian and the Struggle for Physician-Assisted Dying," *Bioethics* 9, no. 1 (Jan. 1995): 62.

42. Kevorkian, *Medicide*, p. 230.

43. Clyde H. Farnsworth, "Tape Recalls A Canadian's Gratitude to Kevorkian," *NYT* (9 May 1996): A17.

44. Bradford Washburn (letter to the editor), "Why can't we be allowed to end life peacefully?" *BG* (16 Dec. 1993): 18.

45. [Editorial,] "Why Dr. Kevorkian Was Called In," *NYT* (25 Jan. 1993): A16, made the connection explicit.

46. Kevorkian, *Medicide,* p. 209.

47. Pence, "Kevorkian and the Struggle," *Bioethics:* 69, quoting from *Newsweek* (8 Mar. 1993): 46, 48.

48. "Advice From Dr. Koop," *Parade Mag.* (7 Apr. 1996): 12.

49. The tape was shown on Mike Wallace's *60 Minutes* program (22 Nov. 1998).

50. Legal and financial considerations both played a role in keeping Kevorkian at home, as becomes evident from a number of comments he makes in *Medicide.*

51. The *NYT* declared "his idiosyncratic crusade has actually begun to hurt the cause he supports." [Editorial,] "Jail Time for Dr. Kevorkian," *NYT* (15 Apr. 1999): A26.

52. Tom L. Beauchamp, ed., "Introduction," *Intending Death: The Ethics of Assisted Suicide and Euthanasia* (Upper Saddle River, N. J.: Prentice Hall, 1996), p. 18.

53. Geoffrey Fieger, personal communication.

54. See Richard Moran and Joseph Ellis, "From the Death Penalty to Euthanasia: The Strange Odyssey of Doctor Jack Kevorkian," *The World & I* (Jan. 1995): 425–31.

55. See Kevorkian, *Medicide,* pp. 182–84.

56. Kevorkian is right. There is historical precedent for some aspects of his views on this topic; he cites German and Armenian medical journals to make his point. But he missed an opportunity to shore up this position when he failed to uncover George M. Shrady quoting (with apparent approval) from an article in the *Journal of Comparative Medicine* a suggestion that the only way to settle whether "man can be infected by the milk or flesh of tuberculous cattle" is to "experiment . . . upon criminals condemned to death." See Shrady's journal, *Medical Record* 19 (19 Mar. 1881): 323.

57. Kevorkian, *Medicide,* p. 183.

58. Quill, "Death and Dignity," *NEJM:* 691–94.

59. Kevorkian, *Medicide,* p. 205. Kevorkian failed to include the subtitle "A Second Look" in his footnote (p. 250n100), raising the question whether he even knew about an earlier article by some of the same doctors, on the same theme, with the same title (minus the subhead). See Sidney H. Wanzer, S. James Adelstein, Ronald E. Cranford, et al., "The Physician's Responsibility Toward Hopelessly Ill Patients," *NEJM* 310, no. 15 (12 Apr. 1984): 955-59, and Sidney H. Wanzer, Daniel D. Federman, S. James Adelstein, et al., "The Physician's Responsibility Toward Hopelessly Ill Patients: A Second Look," *NEJM* 320, no. 13 (30 Mar. 1989): 844–49.

60. Gary E. McCuen, *Doctor Assisted Suicide and the Euthanasia Movement* (Hudson, Wisc.: GEM Publications, 1994).

61. "Dr. Death Strikes Again," *Time* (4 Nov. 1991): 78. Reprinted as a case study ("Assisted Suicide: The Case of Dr. Kevorkian") in Steven Jay Gold, ed., *Moral Controversies* (Belmont, Calif.: Wadsworth, 1993), pp. 187–88.

62. Marilyn Webb, *The Good Death: The New American Search to Reshape the End of Life* (New York: Bantam Books, 1997), pp. 321–60 and generally.

63. One example is the large photo that accompanied Daniel Callahan's "Trying to make peace with human mortality," *BG* (22 Dec. 1991): A22.

64. See *BG* (5 Apr. 1997): A3; the photo was also in the *NYT* (5 Apr. 1997): 12.

65. *BG* (2 Apr. 1996): 3 (photo), 8 ("Kevorkian dresses as Jefferson at new trial").

66. "Kevorkian Mocks Assisted-Suicide Prosecution" was the caption under the picture, published probably shortly prior to the trial that began 1 April 1996, after Kevorkian was charged with assisting in two suicides of non-terminal patients five years earlier.

67. *BG* (5 Mar. 1996): 4 and *NYT* (7 May 1996): A15, respectively.

68. "There has never—truthfully—been anyone like me," Fieger is quoted as saying. We are told "he is everywhere . . . savaging opponents . . . writing furious columns . . . flooding the airwaves." Jack Lessenberry, "Dr. Kevorkian's keeper," *BG* (29 Aug. 1996): D1, D4.

69. Iver Peterson, "In One Doctor's Way of Life, a Way of Death," *NYT* (21 May 1995): 14.

70. "Kevorkian Videotape to Show Patient Dying," *NYT* (20 Nov. 1998): A18.

71. Robert A. Sirico, "Terminal TV," *NYT* (25 Nov. 1998): A27; see also "Kevorkian Videotape," *NYT*: A18.

72. Pam Belluck, "Prosecutor to Weigh Possibility of Charging Kevorkian," *NYT* (23 Nov. 1998): A12.

73. Constance E. Putnam, "Confusion over Kevorkian's Killing," *Concord [Mass.] Journal* (3 Dec. 1998): 6.

74. Raja Mishra, "A study of deaths raises questions on Kevorkian image," *BG* (7 Dec. 2000): A3.

75. Humphry and Clement, *Freedom,* Appendix B: "Laws on Physician-Assisted Suicide in the United States," p. 117. They give as their source the "National Conference on State Legislatures, November 1997."

76. Ronald Dworkin, *Life's Dominion: An Argument About Abortion, Euthanasia, and Individual Freedom* (New York: Knopf, 1993), pp. 4, 183.

77. Derek Humphry, "Assisted suicide law passes in Oregon: now make it work," *ERGO!* (newsletter), no. 1 (Nov. 1994): 1.

78. See William McCall, "Judge rules against Ore. suicide law," *BG* (4 Aug. 1995): 1, 15; "Judge Strikes Down Oregon's Suicide Law," *NYT* (4 Aug. 1995): A15. See also Charles H. Baron, Clyde Bergstresser, Dan W. Brock, et al., "A Model State Act to Authorize and Regulate Physician-Assisted Suicide," *Harvard Jrnl. of Legislation* 33, no. 1 (Winter 1996): 14. The authors' proposal for legislation in Massachusetts was similar in several respects to the Oregon Act.

79. Carey Goldberg, "Oregon Braces for New Fight On Helping the Dying to Die," *NYT* (16 June 1997): A15.

80. Gail Kinsey Hall, "[Governor John] Kitzhaber supports assisted suicide," *Sunday Oregonian* (3 Aug. 1997): A20.

81. Joan Woolfrey, "What Happens Now? Oregon and Physician-Assisted Suicide," *HCR* 28, no. 3 (May-June 1998): 9.

82. See, e.g., "In Oregon, legal doctor-assisted suicide may face federal

obstacles," *BG* (12 Apr. 1998): A13; Neil A. Lewis, "Reno Lifts Barrier To Oregon's Law On Aided Suicide," *NYT* (6 June 1998): A1, A7; also, Adam Pertman, "Bills aim to disarm Oregon law on suicide," *BG* (7 Oct. 1998): A1, A19.

83. Earlier, in the summer of 1996, Australia's Northwest Territory passed a law legalizing physician-assisted suicide; on September 22, 1996, the first patient was assisted to his death. Only two more deaths followed before the law was repealed in 1997, and thus there is little to be learned from the Australian experience. See "Australian doctors are asked to help in an assisted suicide," *BG* (4 July 1996): 8; "Australian Man First in World To Die With Legal Euthanasia," *NYT* (26 Sept. 1996): A5; and Seth Mydans, "Assisted Suicide: Australia Faces a Grim Reality," *NYT* (2 Feb. 1997): 3. Australia's euthanasia debate was later back in the news when a televised ad "in which a terminally ill woman pleads to die" was aired on March 16, 1999. See "TV plea rekindles Australia euthanasia debate," *BG* (18 Mar. 1999): A21. Late in 2001, the debate flared once more when a doctor "accused of murdering a dying patient was acquitted" not long before a survey was published "indicating that many Australian surgeons have hastened death for the terminally ill." See John Shaw, "Australian Doctors Admit Helping Patients Die," *NYT* (3 Dec. 2001): A10.

84. Timothy Egan, "No One Rushing in Oregon To Use a New Suicide Law," *NYT* (15 Mar. 1998): 18, also his "First Death Under an Assisted-Suicide Law," *NYT* (26 Mar. 1998): A14.

85. Sam Howe Verhovek, "Legal Suicide Has Killed 8, Oregon Says," *NYT* (18 Aug. 1998): A16.

86. "Oregon suicide-law study finds no rush to end lives," *BG* (18 Feb. 1999): A3. In 2002, it was reported that only half of the "44 terminally ill patients who had received prescriptions for lethal medication" in the past year ("the most since the law took effect in 1997") had used the drugs. Sam Howe Verhovek, "As Suicide Approvals Rise In Oregon, Half Go Unused," *NYT* (7 Feb. 2002): A16. Oregon remained the only state to permit physician-assisted suicides when the state Senate in Hawaii "rejected a House-passed bill to have Hawaii join Oregon" in legalizing this form of physician-aid-in-dying. The rejected bill was modeled after the Oregon statute. See "Lawmakers reject assisted suicides," *BG* (3 May 2002): A2.

87. "Oregon suicide-law study," *BG:* A3.

88. Arthur E. Chin, Katrina Hedberg, Grant K. Higginson, and David W. Fleming, "Legalized Physician-Assisted Suicide in Oregon—the First Year's Experience," *NEJM* 340, no. 7 (18 Feb. 1999): 582.

89. Hannah Davidson, ed., *Improvements in End-of-Life Care Surrounding Passage of the Oregon Death With Dignity Act* (Portland, Ore.: Oregon Death With Dignity Legal Defense and Education Center [*www.dwd.org*], Oct. 2000): 29.

90. Linda Ganzini, Heidi D. Nelson, Terri A. Schmidt, et al., "Physicians' Experiences with the Oregon Death with Dignity Act," *NEJM* 342, no. 8 (24 Feb. 2000): 557–63.

91. Linda Ganzini, Heidi D. Nelson, Melinda A. Lee, et al., "Oregon Physicians' Attitudes and Experiences Around End-of-Life Care Since Passage of the Oregon Death with Dignity Act," *JAMA* 285, no. 18 (9 May 2001): 2363–69. Some of this information I reported (with commentary) in "New Information on 'Death with Dignity,'" *HCR* 31, no. 4 (July-Aug. 2001): 8.

92. Timothy Quill, personal communication.

93. Susan H. Tolle, "Care of the Dying: Clinical and Financial Lessons from the Oregon Experience," *Ann. of Int. Med.* 128, no. 7 (1 Apr. 1996): 567. A National Hospice Organization newsletter article reported, however, that a study of patients dying in Oregon hospitals showed "an increase in families' reports of their loved ones' pain levels, starting late in 1997" and added that Tolle had "suggested that it may be related to increased publicity about physician-assisted suicide." "News in Hospice's Environment," *NewsLine* 9, no. 2 (1 Feb. 1999): 6.

94. Daniel Labby, personal communication.

95. William L. Toffler, "Oregon Health Plan devalues lives," *Sunday Oregonian* (4 Oct. 1998): G5.

96. Woolfrey, "What Happens Now?" *HCR:* 11.

97. Dan Eggen and Ceci Connolly, "Ashcroft blocks Oregon assisted-suicide law," *BG* (7 Nov. 2001): A2.

98. See, e.g., the exchange on "Death with Dignity" between Greg Eddleston and Richard Horton in "Letters," *The New York Review* (12 Apr. 2001): 89.

99. Joanne Lynn, "President's Letter—Good News! How Outrage Prompted System Change in Oregon," *ABCD Exchange* 4, no. 5/6 (May/June 2001): 5.

100. Ronald Dworkin, "Sex, Death, and the Courts," *The New York Review* (8 Aug. 1996): 44. See also Ronald Dworkin, Thomas Nagel, Robert Nozick, et al., "Assisted Suicide: The Philosophers' Brief," *The New York Review* (27 Mar. 1997): 41–47.

101. See Robert A. Burt, "The Supreme Court Speaks: Not Assisted Suicide but a Constitutional Right to Palliative Care," *NEJM* 357, no. 17 (23 Oct. 1997): 1234–36; and David Orentlicher, "The Supreme Court and Physician-Assisted Suicide: Rejecting Assisted Suicide but Embracing Euthanasia," *NEJM* 357, no. 17 (23 Oct. 1997): 1236–39.

102. Linda Greenhouse, "Court, 9–0, Upholds State Laws Prohibiting Assisted Suicide," *NYT* (27 June 1997): A1.

103. Timothy Quill, personal communication.

104. *Washington v. Glucksberg,* 521 U.S. 702 (1997), at 735.

105. Anthony Deutsch, "Dutch legalize euthanasia," *BG* (11 Apr. 2001): A9. See also Marlise Simons, "Dutch Becoming First Nation to Legalize Assisted Suicide," *NYT* (29 Nov. 2000): A3. Dutch Senate *Handelingen 2000–2001* nr. 27, Eerste Kamer, p. 1295. For the Dutch newspaper account of the lower house vote making Holland "the first country in the world to legalize euthanasia," see *http://www.nvve.nl/informatie/NRC29-11-00.htm,* the Web site of the Dutch euthanasia society (*Nederlandse Vereniging voor Vrijwillige Euthanasie* [NVVE]). See also "Assisted suicides driven by loss of self," *BG* (7 Aug. 2001): C3. For the announcement of the act finally taking effect, see "Dutch Legalize Euthanasia, The First Such National Law," *NYT* (1 Apr. 2002): A9. On 16 May 2002, Belgium "became the second country after the Netherlands to decriminalize euthanasia when the lower house of Parliament adopted a bill giving patients the right to die. After two days of debate, the lower chamber passed the measure by a vote of 86 to 51, with 10 abstentions. The result was widely expected after approval by the Senate in October [2001]." The Belgian law, under consideration for more than a year, was drawn up very much along the lines of the Dutch legislation. *International*

Herald Tribune (17 May 2002): p. 1. See also "La Belgique s'apprête à autoriser l'euthanasie," *Le Temps [Geneva]* (15 May 2002): 42.

106. John Griffiths, Alex Bood, and Heleen Weyers, *Euthanasia & Law in the Netherlands* (Amsterdam: Amsterdam University Press, 1998), p. 18. These authors were not the first to point out that this fact is widely misunderstood. See M.A.M. de Wachter, "Active Euthanasia in the Netherlands," *JAMA* 267, no. 23 (15 Dec. 1989): 3316, and de Wachter, "Euthanasia in the Netherlands," *HCR* 22, no. 2 (Mar.-Apr. 1992): 23–30. I rely heavily on the discussion by Griffiths, Bood, and Weyers for much of what follows in my text.

107. For descriptions of some cases and outcomes, see under "General information about the NVVE" at *http://www.nvve.nl/english/info/jurisprudence.htm*.

108. Ellen Goodman, "'The Dutch way' on euthanasia," *BG* (17 Apr. 1997): A19; "'Dying is not so terrible,'" *BG* (20 Apr. 1997): F7; and "Euthanasia as an option," *BG* (24 Apr. 1997): A27.

109. Goodman, "Euthanasia as an option," *BG:* A27.

110. Griffiths, Bood, and Weyers, *Euthanasia & Law*, p. 111.

111. The "Commission Appointed to Carry out Research Concerning Medical Practice in Connection with Euthanasia" (*Commissie Onderzoek Medische Praktijk inzake Euthanasie*), established by the Second Chamber of Parliament 1989–1990, is regularly referred to by the name of its chairman, J. Remmelink. Griffiths, Bood, and Weyers, *Law & Euthanasia*, p. 77 and 77n108.

112. Griffiths, Bood, and Weyers, *Euthanasia & Law*, p. 132. For a criticism of the idea that ending a patient's life should be considered "normal medical practice," see Henk A.M.J. ten Have and Jos V. M. Welie, "Euthanasia: Normal Medical Practice?" *HCR* 22, no. 2 (Mar.-Apr. 1992): 34–38.

113. Goodman, "'Dutch way,'" *BG:* A17.

114. Griffiths, Bood, and Weyers, *Euthanasia & Law*, p. 16n4.

115. Griffiths, Bood, and Weyers, *Euthanasia & Law*, p. 16.

116. Griffiths, Bood, and Weyers, *Euthanasia & Law*, p. 16n4.

117. Griffiths, Bood, and Weyers, *Euthanasia & Law*, p. 24.

118. Griffiths, Bood, and Weyers, *Euthanasia & Law*, pp. 28n26, 27.

119. Griffiths, Bood, and Weyers, *Euthanasia & Law*, p. 25n19.

120. Carlos Gomez, *Regulating Death: Euthanasia and the Case of the Netherlands* (New York: Free Press, 1991), pp. 22–25, 103, 104. The book is critiqued in John Keown, "On Regulating Death," *HCR* 22, no. 2 (Mar.-Apr. 1992): 39–43.

121. Gomez, *Regulating Death*, pp. 128, 127–28, 136.

122. Herbert Hendin, "Dying of Resentment," *NYT* (21 Mar. 1996): A25.

123. Herbert Hendin, *Seduced by Death: Doctors, Patients and the Dutch Cure* (New York: Norton, 1997), pp. 13, 11.

124. Hendin, *Seduced*, pp. 134, 161, 214.

125. Griffiths, Bood, and Weyers, *Euthanasia & Law*, pp. 25n15, 26.

126. Gerrit van der Wal, *Euthansie en hulp bij zelfdoding door huisartsen [Euthanasia and Suicide with Assistance from Family Doctors]* (Rotterdam: WYT Uitgeefgroep, 1992), p. 123. I am indebted to Ingrid Fischer-van Houte for helping confirm some of my translations from the Dutch.

127. Derek Humphry (letter to the editor), "It's Over, Debbie," *JAMA* 259, no. 14 (8 Apr. 1988): 2096.

128. *"Euthanasie en hulp bij zelfdoding komen dus lang niet zo frequent voor als lange tijd, vooral ook in het buitenland, is gedacht,"* and *"Het is heel goed mogelijk de kwaliteit van het medisch-technisch-euthanatisch handelen te verbeteren"*; van der Wal, *Euthanasie*, pp. 135, 137.

129. The Remmelink Commission's figure of 1,000 cases of non-voluntary euthanasia was reached without distinguishing among family doctors, specialists, and nursing-home physicians (*"geen onderscheid . . . tussen huisartsen, specialisten en verpleeghuisartsen"*); van der Wal, *Euthanasie*, p. 127.

130. See again van der Wal, *Euthanasie*, p. 127 (where he quotes Paul J. van der Maas, Johannes J. M. van Delden, and Loes Pijnenborg, *Medische beslissingen rond het levenseinde* [*Medical Decisions at the End of Life*] ('s Gravenhage: SDU Uitgeverij, 1991), and p. 128.

131. Gerrit van der Wal and P. J. van der Maas, *Euthanasie en andere medische beslissingen rond het levenseinde* [*Euthanasia and Other Medical Decisions at the End of Life*] (The Hague: SDU, 1996).

132. Daniel Callahan, "Trying to make peace with human mortality," *BG* (22 Dec. 1991): A22.

133. Griffiths, Bood, and Weyers, *Euthanasia & Law*, p. 31n4. On the other hand, ending their book with a discussion of whether euthanasia law is "exportable," they observe that perhaps "the most valuable lesson to be drawn from the Dutch experience" is "the quality of the Dutch public discussion itself," p. 305.

134. Herbert Cohen and Timothy Quill also both cite Battin as the most authoritative commentator on this issue, and I have remarked on the way Griffiths, Bood, and Weyers praise her work.

135. Margaret Pabst Battin, "A Dozen Caveats Concerning the Discussion of Euthanasia in the Netherlands," in her *The Least Worst Death: Essays in Bioethics on the End of Life* (New York: Oxford University Press, 1994), pp. 132–33, 135–36, 139–41.

136. Margaret Pabst Battin, "Should We Copy the Dutch? The Netherlands' Practice of Voluntary Active Euthanasia as a Model for the United States," in Robert I. Misbein, ed., *Euthanasia: The Good of the Patient, the Good of Society* (Frederick, Md.: University Publishing Group, 1992), pp. 101, 102.

137. Based on an interview conducted in Amsterdam, June 15, 1998 (and thus prior to the legalization of euthanasia in 2001).

138. Hendin, *Seduced*, pp. 52–53.

139. Paul Wilkes, "The Next Pro-Lifers," *NYT Mag.* (21 July 1996): 26.

140. Ludovic Kennedy, *Euthanasia: The Good Death* (London: Chatto & Windus, 1990), p. 45. Both this quotation and the interview on which my Profile of Cohen is based came prior to the change in Dutch law.

141. See Conference Proceedings, *Whose Death is it Anyway? Medical decisions at the end of life*, Bath, England (World Federation of Right to Die Societies, 10th International Conference, 1994), p. 70.

142. Bert Keizer, *Dancing with Mister D: Notes on Life and Death* (New York: Talese/Doubleday, 1997).

143. Daniel Callahan, *What Kind of Life? The Limits of Medical Progress* (New York: Simon & Schuster, 1990), pp. 144, 145.

144. See Daniel Callahan, *The Troubled Dream of Life: Living with Mortality* (New York: Simon & Schuster, 1993), pp. 40–42.

145. See Jane E. Seymour, "Revisiting medicalisation and 'natural' death," *Soc. Sci. & Med.* 49, no. 5 (Sept. 1999): 691–704.

146. Callahan, *Kind of Life*, p. 236.

147. A classic story is that of Dr. John Bodkin Adams, in England (in 1956), told by the judge in whose court the doctor was acquitted. If Adams "really had an honest belief in easing suffering," the judge later said, he "was on the right side of the law; if his purpose was simply to finish life, he was not." Patrick Devlin, *Easing the Passing: The Trial of Dr. John Bodkin Adams* (London: Bodley Head, 1985), p. 209.

148. Ruth Lewshenia Kopp (with Stephen Sorenson), *Encounter with Terminal Illness* (Grand Rapids, Mich.: Zondervan Publishing, 1980), p. 86.

149. Daniel Goleman, "Doctors Find Comfort Is a Potent Medicine," *NYT* (26 Nov. 1991): C1.

150. Robert Pear, "Doctors Say H.M.O.'s Limit What They Can Tell Patients," *NYT* (21 Dec. 1995): A1.

151. Bob Herbert, "Hidden Agenda," *NYT* (15 July 1996): A13.

152. Francis Weaver, "People have a right to decide medical fate," and Sylvia Gerhard, "Finding comfort by gaining control" (letters to the editor), *BG* (8 Apr. 1996): 18.

153. N. C. Webb (letter to the editor), "Death, dignity and the doctor," *BG* (2 Apr. 1996): 18.

154. Francis D. Moore, "Prolonging Life, Permitting Life to End," *Harvard Mag.* 97, no. 6 (July-Aug. 1995): 47.

155. Based on an interview conducted at Genesee Hospital in Rochester, New York, November 10, 1998.

156. Jane Gross, "Doctor at Center of Supreme Court Case on Assisted Suicide," *NYT* (2 Jan. 1997): B1.

157. Timothy E. Quill, *A Midwife Through the Dying Process: Stories of Healing & Hard Choices at the End of Life* (Baltimore: Johns Hopkins University Press, 1996).

158. Gross, "Doctor," *NYT*: B1.

159. Gross, "Doctor," *NYT*: B1.

160. Quill, "Death and Dignity," *NEJM*: 694.

161. Richard M. Doerflinger (letter to the editor), "Slippery Slope in Action," *NYT* (7 Jan. 1997): A16. The *NYT* identified Doerflinger as associate director for policy, Secretariat for Pro-Life Activities, National Conference of Catholic Bishops.

5

Putting Principles into Practice

Die allerletzte Pein ist, glaub ich, ärger nicht,
Als leben müssen, todt seyn wollen und nicht können.
[There can be no worse pain, I believe,
Than having to live, when you want to die and cannot.]
—Simon Dach[1]

In this chapter I will examine some of the principles most commonly invoked in discussions about decision-making at the end of life and then present some steps one might take while applying those principles to the contentious issues raised so far. I will do this by presenting model arguments as examples of how one might test one's own commitment to a particular position. We will then look at how using principles and arguments can help us understand the shape and direction of our lives. Finally, we will look at how discourse on the subject of death and dying—especially between doctors and patients—can also increase that understanding.

USING EXTERNAL PRINCIPLES FOR EVALUATION

In order to judge whether a health-care system (or at least that part of it having to do with the care of dying patients) meets acceptable standards, we need to know what the standards are. Identifying and clarifying those standards is not easy. Nonetheless, various individuals and institutions within the health-care world have done just that. A set of principles proposed by the Hastings Center (in 1987) will serve present purposes well.[2] (Others have previously identified this set of principles as the "most prominent" among "a number of distinct ethical values" that need to be considered.[3])

As specified in the report from the Hastings Center, the ethical values that underlie treatment decisions are these: patient self-determination (individual autonomy), patient well-being (beneficence), the ethical integrity of health-care professionals (professional integrity), and justice or equity.[4] Let's examine these, one at a time. (We will see that there is considerable overlap.)

"Individual autonomy" or "patient self-determination"[5] means at the very least that patients should be allowed to make their own, informed decisions. In today's climate, especially, this should not be problematic; the importance of autonomy is not a new idea. Philosopher Elizabeth L. Beardsley, for example, insisted some thirty years ago that the "injunction against violations of autonomy is so basic that it can appropriately occupy a place at or near the foundations of any set of moral principles; . . . many of the interesting problems involve decisions about when it may be justifiably overridden."[6] But although we would like to be able to assume, today, that autonomy for patients entails patients being able to count on their physicians to neither condescend nor behave paternalistically, there are difficulties. For example, physician Mark Siegler, in an exploration of "the limits of autonomy,"[7] stressed that there is a wide variety of factors influencing physicians' clinical decisions; the patient's autonomy might not be the chief one.

Philosopher Bruce L. Miller has made relying on a principle of autonomy even more difficult, arguing that truly autonomous decisions have four independent dimensions. They must be "free actions," they must have "authenticity," and they must exhibit both "effective deliberation" and "moral reflection." When physicians are in doubt about whether a patient's preferred decision is autonomous in all four of those ways, they may (according to Miller) override the patient's decision. The ground for doing so—what makes it permissible—is that the decision was (by Miller's criteria) not truly autonomous. Hence the patient's right to autonomy would not have been violated. Miller's conclusion is troubling. Decisions to override are not necessarily paternalistic (and not all paternalism is unjustified or otherwise wrong, anyway), but Miller leaves all the wiggle room on the physician's side. If physicians are permitted in this manner to override patients' preferred decisions, the opportunity certainly exists for unwarranted paternalism to creep in.[8]

"Patient autonomy" today undeniably implies that patients must give their informed consent before health-care decisions that affect them are carried out. Further, as we saw in Chapter 3, the right of patients to refuse treatments they do not want, even if they are life-saving treatments, has long been established; responding to patients' wishes to forgo life-sustaining or life-extending treatment has gradually become less controversial. As a result, "physicians have begun to question whether they must always comply with requests to continue or limit such treatment, even when they disagree with the rationale or intent of those requests"; further, "ethicists have responded by reexamining the line between patient autonomy and physician authority."[9]

One problem is that the view physicians and patients have on the appropriateness or the possible futility of a treatment may be in conflict. I mentioned when discussing futility earlier that some physicians believe "futility is a professional judgment that takes precedence over patient autonomy."[10] Although the same authors go on to acknowledge that "potential for abuse is present,"[11] others argue that we have to be careful not to lean too far in the direction of protecting patients' rights if it means we are going to ignore physicians' judgments. Donald J. Murphy, for example, insists that advocating "a unilateral decision by the health care team . . . can be criticized as paternalistic. [But s]ince paternalism is ultimately based on the ethical principle of beneficence, . . . paternalism may be justified in some situations."[12] Stuart J. Youngner, however, accuses Murphy of lapsing "into an outdated (but perhaps yearned for) notion of paternalism," and says that his "proposal is a regressive step. Under the guise of medical expertise and concern for proper resource allocation, it encourages physicians to substitute their own value judgments for those of their patients."[13]

Implementing "beneficence" is—from the doctor's perspective—all part of what is involved in making medical decisions (even though those decisions may conflict with patient autonomy). That is just what doctors do. Sometimes expressed more narrowly as "promoting patient welfare,"[14] beneficence means that the well-being of the patient is what should guide the physician's actions and help determine the appropriate treatments, medications, and procedures. (This is what Miller would say occasionally justifies overriding a patient's expressed wishes.) But this is not a very precise principle. What exactly counts as benefiting the patient is not always clear. And if doctor and patient disagree, whose idea of benefit should take precedence? As we have seen, a central feature of the whole Hospice vs. Hemlock debate rests on how this question is answered: Can a doctor helping a patient die possibly be seen as benefiting that patient?

It is also exceedingly easy for those in a position to make decisions to become confused about the principles of decision-making. We pretend we are "complying . . . with the wishes of the patients," making a "substituted judgment," when we are actually giving "mere lip service" to that principle, as law professor Charles Baron has pointed out.[15] A decision in favor of death over PVS (for someone else) is apt rather to be made on "best-interests" grounds, like deciding that a child's "getting a shot" (which *hurts*) is in that child's best interests. Even adults have difficulty with this kind of idea, that there is benefit in unpleasant-tasting medicines or capsules so large they are difficult to swallow, never mind the indignity and discomfort of being subjected to a sigmoidoscopy or having one's stomach pumped. The benefits of these (and worse) discomforts and inconveniences are rarely intuitively obvious. Still, some things are clear: Patient welfare (beneficence) surely rules out, for instance, experimenting on patients without their permission when there is no expectation that the experiment will do the patients any good (and where, as in some cases, steps known to be beneficial are deliberately not taken). It should also rule out refusing to treat pain aggressively for fear of a malpractice suit if the dosage proves lethal. Whether being helped to die is beneficial is a considerably trickier matter to evaluate.

The "ethical integrity of health-care professionals" or the "integrity of the [medical] profession" is another complex principle that lacks precision.[16] Presumably it means something like this: Health-care professionals should neither be required to do, nor do of their own volition, anything that is not consistent with maintaining their integrity as members of the health-care profession to which they belong. For some, the most obvious example of how doctors stay true to the integrity of their profession is for them to take seriously the absolute prohibition against killing: "Doctors mustn't kill," we hear on many sides.

Another superficially obvious part of what it means to maintain the integrity of the profession is to follow such precepts as "cure where possible" and "care for by alleviating suffering when cure is no longer an option." (The close relationship between "beneficence" and at least some features of the "integrity of the profession" becomes evident here.) Yet we do not necessarily know, or agree about, what is "possible" with respect to cures. Further, what counts as "suffering" is not the same for all people, nor does everyone agree completely about how to alleviate suffering most effectively. Despite the best efforts of the best palliative-care physicians, it still seems to be true that there will be times when a given patient's suffering cannot be adequately relieved or removed. That applies to psychic and social as well as somatic pain. Timothy Quill reports that some "patients must often make very difficult choices on a daily basis between pain and sedation," and that for "a few patients, even those on hospice programs, the end can be agonizing and completely out of their control."[17]

Similar disagreements arise over what content should be included in "integrity of the profession": truth-telling? doctor-patient confidentiality? a duty to treat? a willingness to make sacrifices for one's patients or run personal health (and other) risks? It is not enough to say that doctors should act like doctors, be the best they can be, not cut corners or let the other members of their profession down, and so on—though considerations such as these are surely connected with the idea of the integrity of the profession. Moreover, as physician Marcia Angell has pointed out, the latter years of the twentieth century brought new tensions between "doctors' traditional public responsibilities" and "their primary role of serving the medical needs of their individual patients."[18] In other words, just as what it means to be a health-care professional changes, what it means to uphold the integrity of the profession is constantly evolving.

"Justice" appropriately comes into play as a principle (or set of principles) in health care, because we see health care as one of the societal goods to be shared—distributed—among those who need it. But figuring out exactly what justice in health care requires of us is by no means simple, as philosopher Norman Daniels has amply demonstrated in his book *Just Health Care* (1985), devoted to precisely this issue.[19] To suggest that we look at justice as fairness is to follow an intuitive sense that many of us share; the basic idea of fairness is crucial to the common understanding of justice (its best current development is in the work of philosopher John Rawls[20]). We understand, in other words, that something is not just if it is not fair. Most people would presumably also agree, at least upon reflection, that fairness in health care is determined in part by whether those in need of treatment have fair access to the care and treatment they need. If artificial (and morally irrelevant) barriers are set up so that only certain classes of patients have access to health-care services, or if natural barriers or distinctions that carry no moral weight (such as skin color or sexual orientation) are allowed to interfere with access, fundamental unfairness will almost certainly result. If I am unable to get the health care I need when you can get it for the same needs, that is fundamentally unfair.

A just health-care system will focus more on fairness than on equality (we may not have equal needs). That means the system will treat us in proportion to our needs, so that we arrive in as nearly the same place as possible. The way Rawls expresses this is to say that what justice requires is that each of us must be guaranteed "fair equality of opportunity." The point of such a fair equality of opportunity, Daniels says, is to enable each of us (to the extent possible) to function within the "normal range of opportunities."[21]

We are now ready to use these principles to make comparative evaluations of Hospice and Hemlock. At the outset, we see that the principle of autonomy creates some tension within Hospice. The strict ideology according to which many Hospice physicians operate often looks like paternalism. When the Hospice philosophy is adhered to in a doctrinaire manner, patients who do not agree with what those in charge think constitutes their well-being may find their autonomy unacceptably undermined. For the patient who subscribes fully and in every particular to the Hospice philosophy presumably no problem arises, and there is no obvious loss of autonomy. But we have plenty of anecdotal evidence of instances where a patient receiving Hospice care is *not* in complete agreement with all aspects of the Hospice approach.

As for autonomy and Hemlock, there is a very good match. Indeed, the whole thrust of the Hemlock philosophy is that individual patients have the right to make their own decisions about what is in their best interest (and what constitutes their well-being). Hemlock philosophy rests heavily on the precept that respect for persons requires treating their decisions about their own lives—and deaths—as the decisions of autonomous people. Clearly the principle of autonomy (as most of us would probably interpret it) is salient in Hemlock. If, as Derek Humphry puts it, the right to die is the ultimate civil liberty,[22] then Hemlock is going to support the individual's right to choose without reference to someone else's idea of what that choice ought to be.

When it comes to the principle of beneficence, Hospice certainly seems to earn an extremely high rating. All the Hospice rhetoric (and the activity generated out of that rhetoric) is aimed quite explicitly at taking the best possible care of the patient. The patient's welfare—doing what is good for the patient, doing what is in the patient's best interest—appears to be uppermost. At least two questions need to be raised, however: "Whose definition of what is good for the patient is taken as dispositive?" and "Who decides exactly what is in the patient's best interests?" Debates over whether a "best interests" argument is adequate when deciding on treatment for an incompetent patient illustrate this well. "In practice," we are told, "the 'best interests' of a patient are assumed to coincide with what most 'reasonable persons' would choose in the same circumstances."[23] This assumption seems to me rather to beg the question, however, by blurring the distinction between a "substituted judgment" (which entails making a decision as the other person would) and making a "best interests" argument (which means deciding what is best for that other person). The difference is subtle but important.

Hemlock supporters might also insist that the whole point of their approach is to assure that patients are treated in the way they believe is most conducive to their own welfare. Given room to operate on its own terms, Hemlock certainly aims at beneficence. But notice the shift in point of view. "Beneficence" is generally thought to be a measure of the physician's behavior toward the patient; Hemlock turns that around, saying that Hemlock is beneficent because it leaves room and opportunity for dying persons to act in a way they consider beneficent. Until more laws change, however, it will continue to be difficult for physicians to act on the version of beneficence that dying Hemlock supporters may have in mind. Thus Hemlock claims allegiance to the principle of beneficence but finds itself still trying to create a social and legal climate where its kind of beneficence is available.

For Hospice, the principle of maintaining the integrity of the medical profession by making it absolutely clear that Hospice physicians will not prematurely end their patients' lives (they won't, in other words, "kill"), is key to their basic philosophy. The result is that Hospice simply does not give room for certain kinds of decisions that are open to physicians operating under other principles. (One could here raise the question of the autonomy of the *physician*, and see how well Hospice rates on such a measure—but this would be to change the subject.) In its favor, Hospice can claim to be clear about things that are subject to difficult debate outside its confines, and certainly for some people this is an enormous advantage.

Another potential plus for Hospice is that it sees upholding the integrity of the medical profession (of health professionals in general) as more than just avoiding prohibited activity. For Hospice, just as important as prohibitions like "doctors mustn't kill" are affirmative exhortations: "relieve suffering," "treat the whole patient (psychically, spiritually, and socially as well as somatically)," "support the family of the dying patient as well as the patient." Taken together, the prohibitions and the preachments that go with the Hospice practices and policies are not only clear but possible to interpret with considerable precision. The result is that health-care professionals within Hospice may have a stronger sense of exactly what it means to uphold the integrity of the profession than will some of their colleagues who work outside Hospice. If a statement of rigid principles with which physicians must comply—coupled with a broad interpretation of the physician's responsibilities—is what is wanted, Hospice serves the integrity of the profession very well indeed. As one doctor who has integrated Hospice principles into his practice says,

Palliative care offers several potential solutions to this dilemma. One theme in palliative care is its emphasis on improving communications. Traditionally, physicians are trained to see their interests with patients and families as primarily information-based. Palliative care looks at discussions between clinicians and patients or surrogates as conversations; that is, each party brings to the interaction emotional and personal factors that are crucial to mutual understanding.[24]

I have hinted already at the challenge for health-care professionals who operate according to Hemlock principles rather than Hospice principles. Clarity and absolutes are exactly what they do not have. The central importance of autonomy within the Hemlock framework means that health-care professionals must have a much more flexible sense of what it means to act with integrity. To take an example we have looked at a couple of times already: Most physicians who support Hemlock will subscribe to the principle that doctors mustn't kill. But their desire to give pride of place to autonomy requires a more complex understanding of what it means to help end someone's life than is demanded of Hospice physicians. All concerned may agree that "killing" patients is contrary to upholding the integrity of the profession. But more is needed than a definition of "killing" that can be used in a wide range of circumstances. It is also necessary to balance such norms as "heal the sick (when possible)" and "do no harm," when persisting in the curing mode in fact causes distress, discomfort, or worse, and when refusing to *end* the suffering for the patient may also be a matter of doing harm. Hemlock requires a broader and less rigid understanding of "integrity of the profession" than Hospice does—and that has both advantages and disadvantages.

If we accept the idea of "justice as fairness," Hospice rates very high. Hospice offers equal-opportunity treatment to all comers: The potentially curable are treated no differently—if they do not wish to pursue cure—from those for whom no physical improvements can be expected. But although Hospice is theoretically available to all, in practice it is not. Even the aggressive palliative care that is so centrally a part of Hospice (and increasingly outside Hospice as well) is not everywhere available, as we have seen. Further, although Hospice is supposed to be open to all, it remains in many of its incarnations a strongly Christian foundation and approaches care with a self-conscious focus on religious sensibility or spirituality. Not everyone wants to do the "work" (spiritual, social, familial) at the end of life so central to the Hospice ideal of what it means for patients to have the chance to "live fully until they die." (As Timothy Quill has pointed out, the "ideal" put forward in the "unexpressed 'ideology'" of Hospice is "not for everyone."[25]) Thus whether the care offered by Hospice is truly fair—that is, just—even for those who manage to get access to it is not altogether clear.

Hemlock has its own problems with justice. Central to Hemlock thinking is that dying persons should have the right to die in a time and manner of their own choosing. (For simplicity's sake, leave aside the issue of whether a non-terminal patient who wants to die has the same right as the terminally ill patient.[26]) We can certainly imagine two cases of dying patients alike in every regard except that one has the physical ability requisite to effecting his or her own death (committing suicide), and the other does not. Is a system "just" that does not accommodate the second person as well as the first? Is it fair? The prima facie *un*fairness of such a situation is precisely part of what has pushed some Hemlock supporters (not merely the radical extremists, either) to insist that where there is a right to die there must also be a right to obtain assistance from a willing provider. With this in mind, we can see that Hemlock has some serious problems to face if it is to be judged fully just.

Which comes off better: Hospice or Hemlock? Neither fails utterly on any of the four principles. If Hemlock does better with respect to both beneficence and autonomy, as I believe it does, a case can be made for saying that Hospice does better on integrity of the profession (as that phrase is usually, conservatively, understood). As for justice, both Hospice and Hemlock meet the requirement marginally. In any case, the answer to the question about which rates better will to some extent be a matter for each individual to settle on his or her own (a feature of this whole enterprise to be explored in greater detail shortly).

Let us move now to the second phase of our effort to assess Hospice and Hemlock by using principles as measuring rods. So far we have looked at the application of *externally* determined principles to Hospice and Hemlock; we turn next to look at how one might evaluate Hospice and Hemlock by applying principles *internally* espoused by those movements. Reviewing every operative principle and all possible arguments is a very large task; my aim here is only to illustrate the beginning of the process, the *kind* of effort the task requires.

USING INTERNAL PRINCIPLES FOR EVALUATION

Of course it is possible to state arguments for and against euthanasia, as people do. The danger comes from the tendency either to give very short shrift to the whole process or to expatiate at such length that ordinary readers lose track of what is being argued. An illustration of this can be found in a book on death and dying edited by Tom L. Beauchamp and Seymour Perlin, who list the "pervasive" and "most popular" arguments on euthanasia. Those in favor are arguments from individual liberty, from loss of human dignity, and from the reduction of suffering. Those against are from the sanctity of human life, from probable abuse, from wrong diagnoses and new treatments, and the wedge argument. But the single-paragraph descriptions they give in their introduction do not constitute a set of formal arguments, and they lose the virtue of brevity when they are taken up at article length.[27] Furthermore, as philosopher Dan W. Brock has reminded us, we "often fail to recognize the problematic nature of particular assumptions or views and so fail to subject them to the criticism they deserve."[28]

The importance of uncovering and acknowledging hidden premises and implicit assumptions in our arguments cannot be stressed too much. "It is in our tacit assumptions that we most clearly reveal our working philosophies," Abraham Kaplan said in his remarks summing up a symposium on "The Sanctity of Life" more than three decades ago.[29] We may discover after analyzing our own views that they need to be revised; this is the whole point, it could be said, of engaging in moral reflection in the first place. The most considered judgments we make may turn out not to be quite what we thought they were once we have examined their underpinnings. As John Rawls has pointed out, "even the judgments we take provisionally as fixed points are liable to revision," and "we may want to change our present considered judgments once their regulative principles are brought to light."[30] Though we often act as if our most deeply held moral beliefs are necessary truths, believing them to be so does not make them so. Furthermore, they are much more likely to be contingent truths at best; this is another reason for continuing to explore the roots of our belief systems and for staying open to reflection and revision.

Why is it that a sound argument, easy to follow and to understand, is so rare? For one thing, constructing arguments that are both valid and persuasive is seldom easy. Perhaps not surprisingly, therefore, a lot of the public debate continues to be anything but systematic. As my earlier discussion of Jack Kevorkian was intended to show, it was the flamboyance of his activities that put in front of so many people the question of whether they would want anyone to help them die, and if so who and how. But at least in part because of his dramatic self-promotion, the discussion surrounding his actions was generally more emotional than rational.

We need now to look in a systematic way at the questions of whether Hospice is enough and whether Hemlock is too much. We need to explore the differences in the arguments on which each movement relies. In making those differences explicit—more specifically, in making the underlying claims (the hidden premises) explicit—I have two aims. I hope both to reduce the confusion that arises for casual observers and to establish a model for how to begin investigating other pieces of the complex puzzle that comprises end-of-life decisions.

Hospice and Hemlock, though ostensibly concerned with the same basic issue (how to assure that an individual's dying days are filled with as little misery and as much meaning as possible), generally seem to be at loggerheads. Their respective approaches to the dying process appear incompatible; my aim is to see whether and how a passable bridge between the two can be built. My method will be first to take principles that come out of Hospice and Hemlock literature respectively and then to build arguments by uncovering the hidden premises on which the principles seem to be based.

My strategy has been to isolate two key tenets of "Hospice" and two for "Hemlock." I then formulated those tenets as principles for each of the movements.[31] As we shall see, despite the shared goal of making the dying process as little burdensome as possible, fundamental differences exist between the two approaches. I have formulated the principles in a way that emphasizes the similarities and the dissimilarities between the two movements. Doing this helps make absolutely clear that the differences, which put Hospice and Hemlock at the extreme ends of a continuum, are dramatic and critical.

The two Hospice principles look like this:

P_1 Dying is a natural life-cycle process that ought not necessarily to include suffering, the fear of suffering, or loneliness; no one who does not choose to should have to die alone or in pain.

P$_2$ Affirming life means doing nothing to prolong or delay the dying process; human dignity is maintained by living life fully to the end. ("Hospice care should include nothing that will intentionally either delay *or* hasten the natural dying process" is how I put it earlier.)

The two Hemlock principles look like this:

P$_3$ Everyone has a right to make decisions about when and how to alleviate the pain that may accompany his or her own dying; no one should interfere with an individual's efforts to manage pain or to seek help in its management.

P$_4$ An individual's life is his or her own—and only the individual in question can know when that life has reached its tolerable limits, when the maintenance of personal dignity permits making a choice in favor of death. (Raising the issue of whether there is a "right to do whatever it takes to alleviate unremitting pain" is how I put this earlier.)

The first principle in each pair—Hospice P$_1$, Hemlock P$_3$—deals with basically the same issue, namely pain, and there is a substantial overlap between the two. Closer analysis will reveal that they are by no means identical, however. The emphasis in each is different, and the routes taken to reach the respective positions are not the same.

Far greater differences appear between the second principle in each pair—Hospice P$_2$, Hemlock P$_4$—though both speak to the issue of human dignity. The assertions in each are based on very different ideas of what "dignity" means; as a result, these principles are potentially in serious conflict with each other. Again, and more obviously and importantly than in the case of the first pair, the route to Hospice P$_2$ is not the same as the route to Hemlock P$_4$.

Hence, it is on what we might call "the route taken"—the arguments—that we need to concentrate our deliberations. The first step is to spell out the arguments; the second is to take the differences that emerge and try to find common ground on which to bring the two arguments together if at all possible. The sharpness of this conflict between groups with a shared goal is a large part of what makes it difficult for most people to know what to think, let alone for society as a whole to agree on what is appropriate.

PAIN AND DIGNITY-OF-LIFE ARGUMENTS

Hospice P$_1$, it will be recalled, looks like this: *Dying is a natural life-cycle process that ought not necessarily to include suffering, the fear of suffering, or loneliness; no one who does not choose to should have to die alone or in pain.* Behind that lies a series of premises that constitute the basis of the argument implicitly being made. Those premises and their conclusion must look something like the following:

Dying alone or in pain is unpleasant.

It is undignified (unworthy for human beings) to have to go through this kind of unpleasantness.

It is unnecessary to have to go through this kind of unpleasantness, and those who choose to try to avoid it should not have to put up with it.

As members of a community (the community of human beings, implicit in the sweeping "No one should have to"), we have a collective responsibility to spare each other unpleasantness that is undignified (unworthy of our status as human beings) as much as possible when it is not wanted; especially when the unpleasantness is unnecessary, the burden of that collective responsibility is heavy.

Therefore, steps should be taken to reduce the pain that may accompany the natural life-cycle process of dying for those who wish to have it reduced and to assure that those who are dying are not left alone unless they choose to be.

The conclusion in the final step is essentially equivalent to Hospice principle P_1.

Hemlock P_3 was this: *Everyone has a right to make decisions about when and how to alleviate the pain that may accompany his or her own dying; no one should interfere with an individual's efforts to manage pain or to seek help in its management.* The argument would have to run more or less like this:

Knowledge of and experience in pain control do not rest in the medical establishment alone (witness the successes of faith healing, alternative medicine, New Age holism, etc.).

The medical establishment has in any case manifestly failed to manage pain adequately in every instance (numerous anecdotes testify to this generalization).

Individuals know their own pain limits (toleration level) better than anyone else.

Therefore, individuals should be free to decide for themselves when and what they need in the way of pain medication; the decision should not have to be filtered through anyone else (most especially not through the medical establishment).

The conclusion in step four is more or less equivalent to Hemlock principle P_3.

Similar discrepancies exist between the premises that emerge when we look behind the scenes at the second of the two principles in each movement. Hospice P_2 was this: *Affirming life means doing nothing to prolong or delay the dying process; human dignity is maintained by living life fully to the end.* Here the argument runs as follows:

Life as such is a prime value; dying is a natural life-cycle process, and—accordingly—it should not be interfered with (death will come in its own good time).

We are in any case not masters of our own lives (as is evident from the way the Christian theological basis for much of Hospice thinking—we are God's creation, and we are but stewards of something that belongs to God when we make decisions about our lives—is made explicit in much of the Hospice literature.)

Therefore, it is inappropriate for us to choose to take deliberate action either to prolong or to hasten the end of anyone's life, including our own.

The conclusion in the third step is more or less equivalent to Hospice principle P_2.

Hemlock P_4 was this: *An individual's life is his or her own—and only the individual in question can know when that life has reached its tolerable limits, when the maintenance of personal dignity permits making a choice in favor of death.* And the argument goes like this:

My life is my own.

I know what is (for me) a good (or at least tolerable) life.

No one else is able to make judgments for me on the degree to which my condition fits acceptably within the range of what I consider tolerable.

Therefore, I may do as I please, that is, I have a *right* to make my own choice about when it is appropriate to end my life.

The conclusion in the fourth step is essentially equivalent to Hemlock principle P_4.

THE TRAJECTORY OF A LIFE

What I mean by "the trajectory of a life" is best understood this way: Thinking about the trajectory of one's life means calculating the likely extension of the path(s) one has followed to date, whether by deliberate plan or simply by being caught up in adventitious circumstances. What interests me here is trying to trace a trajectory that results from answering the following types of questions: What sort of person am I? What are the concerns that matter most to me? What kind of a life have I led heretofore?

These are, of course, exceedingly difficult questions to address. Not only will different individuals answer them very differently, but the answers any one person gives will shift over time. Still, some attempt to put the questions into focus will almost certainly make our present task—trying to divine what path it makes the most sense to follow during the dying process—more manageable. Tracing the trajectory of one's life as fully as possible is one way of getting a hint as to what is appropriate when that life comes to an end.

Deciding on the best course of action is so inherently difficult that be-ing able to rule out some of the variables, or at least to recognize them as merely tangential, is bound to help. One way to start would be to make a list of principles like the four guidelines from the Hastings Center dis-cussed earlier and then to try rank-ordering them as to their relative im-portance for us individually. For example: Am I the sort of person for whom increasing the sum total of good in the world is a primary goal? Then "beneficence" might come first. Or am I a person for whom the right to choose is paramount? Then "individual autonomy" would have pride of place. But caution is in order. Just as most of our important rights turn out to be cluster rights, the values expressed by the Hastings Center guide-lines may also have "cluster" qualities to them. (We have already seen how some of them overlap with each other.) It is well within reason, for in-stance, for someone to argue that respect for "individual autonomy" is precisely one feature of what makes up "beneficence," and that thus these two should not be separated. And we have already seen how some people might consider "integrity of the medical profession" to be a combination of beneficence and non-maleficence.

Leaving aside the Hastings Center guidelines, let us tackle the task of judging what kinds of persons we are by another approach. Am I, one might ask oneself, the sort of person concerned to guide my life prima-rily by reference to what the law requires and forbids? Or am I a person for whom commitment to the precepts of a particular religious tradition is the controlling feature of how I choose to act? Am I focused on my own position in society and getting what I consider my due—or am I, in some fundamental way, concerned about the good of society as a whole with-out regard to what may happen to me personally?

The list of such questions could easily be extended, and they admittedly overlap with each other. The result is that the answer to no one of them can tell me with precision what kind of person I am, but each such ques-tion that I *can* answer is another point to be plotted on the curve of my personal trajectory. Gradually, a pattern should begin to emerge that will facilitate the formation of arguments appropriate to my own situation and my own life.

For instance, if religious questions are of primary importance to me, I would want to ask and answer specific questions related to end-of-life decisions, like the following: What does my religion teach about death? Does God alone determine the time of an individual's death, or do I have a right to say or do anything about it? Am I to believe that there is some special spiritual meaning to be attached to the manner in which I die?

Consider on the other hand the possibility that adherence to the law is of the greatest concern to me. My questions might look like this: Does the law permit me to take my own life? Does the law permit someone else to assist me in dying? Do physicians have any special status under the law when it comes to helping people die? In either case, I may need to consider questions connected to some social issues: If physicians were to be allowed to help patients die, would that have a detrimental effect on society? How would it affect the "integrity of the profession"? Should, in other words, physician-aid-in-dying be considered acceptable social policy? Is palliative care available to all who need it and does (or should) this concern me? Is my death really a private matter and not a social one at all?

Answering such questions is fraught with difficulties; figuring out how to deal with one's own dying is challenging for anyone. We each need to get our own priorities straight in order to answer questions like this for ourselves. "Most dying patients do not have a clearly defined route of exit," Timothy Quill tells us.[32] But if we are lucky, as Richard W. Momeyer has tried to show, we will indeed have some "significant choices presented to each of us as to what kind of approach we will individually take to death. And the approach we take to death, not as a matter of psychological necessity or social conditioning but as a function of reflection and the search for self-knowledge, reveals our true selves as clearly as anything can."[33]

The real test, marking whether we have constructed adequate arguments for ourselves, will always be this: Have I examined carefully—carefully enough, as carefully as I can—what is in fact meant by whatever I say or claim to believe? The importance of doing this is apparent when we face the reality that there is not, and never will be, a single "correct" way to approach death. Even those who share a religious heritage that grounds them solidly enough to give clear, indisputable, and identical answers to some of the attendant questions may still find that, because of their individual circumstances, their answers to other relevant questions are not the same. And even those who take their religious arguments very seriously may nevertheless in the end find they have to subordinate the religious arguments to some others when the arguments lead to conflicting conclusions and choices must therefore be made.

Earlier we used model arguments to help uncover hidden assumptions and implicit premises; let's try a similar tactic here. A highly independent and secular individual, to take one possible case, might come up with a first attempt to make decisions based on an underlying argument like this:

I am a free and autonomous person.

Self-determination is a central feature of being a free and autonomous person.

Self-determination includes the right to determine the time and manner of one's own death, other things being equal.

Therefore, I should not have to tolerate any (unreasonable) interference with my decisions on matters having to do with my death.

On the other hand, a deeply religious person might argue like this:

Human life is granted each of us in trust from God.

All decisions about how I live—and that includes how I approach death—are to be made with God's plan for that life in mind.

My own wishes and desires are secondary in the greater scheme of God's plans.

Therefore, I must submit to God's will (as manifest in the course of nature) when it comes time for me to die; I have no basis for making any decision in this regard on my own.

Both these arguments (which loosely approximate what one might expect from Hemlock and Hospice supporters respectively) are rather crude, but they suffice to show what different foundations the advocates of one or the other of these arguments are likely to stand on as they contemplate end-of-life decisions. Noting this—indeed, making a point of trying to understand those whose conclusions are at odds with our own—may help further clarify and strengthen our own convictions. As Daniel C. Maguire once said, "It is fair to say that if you do not know the objections to your position, you do not know your position."[34] Understanding different positions (not merely understanding that differences exist) is critical to grasping why people disagree so strongly about how life should end. If we are willing to try to understand each other as we strive to remain true to ourselves, we have a chance at finding common ground. What turns out to be shared could be, for example, a belief in the sanctity of life or a conviction that death should not be painful or lonely for those who do not wish it to be.

DOCTOR-PATIENT DIALOGUE

After all this critical introspection is said and done, however, a major task remains. No matter how clear we are in our own minds about what we believe and what the supporting arguments are, there is still the issue of what we can expect from our physicians. Once we know what choices we want (or intend) to make for ourselves, how do we see to it that our choices are not overridden?

Of course we might not be in a position to execute our choices. Any one of us might die suddenly in circumstances that offer no opportunity for our views on the matter to be brought to bear. In this day of modern technological wonders and apparent medical miracles, however, we are more likely to find ourselves (or others about whom we care) in a situation where we can influence how death comes. Modern death tends to be medically managed, and the dying process—as we are frequently reminded in reports of formal studies, personal essays, and articles in almost any newspaper we pick up—is likely to be the object of a great deal of manipulation. Precisely because so many aspects of the dying process frequently *can* be arranged, it behooves us as rational beings to take all possible steps to become clear not only about our own views, but also about those of our physicians. At the very least, this means talking to our physicians to find out what their views are. And lest the "manipulation" or what is "arranged" be totally out of keeping with our deeply held views (off the track of our own particular life's trajectory), we should want to be clear that what we proclaim to be our beliefs rest on arguments whose premises we can accept. This is the significance of the sketchy samples of arguments proposed above.

But how to talk with the doctors? Discussions about death and dying have increasingly included analyses of the doctor-patient relationship; some of what has been said is discouraging. I have argued elsewhere that "[r]ational decision-making takes both time and talk, whoever engages in it; shared decision-making most certainly requires time for shared talk—though we must not pretend that time for talk (communication) is a sufficient condition for shared decision-making."[35]

Even extensive efforts to improve communication between physicians and patients do not necessarily yield the desired results, as the widely reported "SUPPORT" study showed. A complex, controlled trial aimed at improving care for seriously ill (hospitalized) patients, its second phase involved testing carefully researched interventions (outgrowths of the first phase of the study) that were intended to improve communication between doctors and their dying patients.[36] And when the best possible changes in doctor-patient relations are made, they may still not yield perfect results. For starters, more *talk* between concerned parties does not guarantee "communication" in any very meaningful sense of the word. Also, building adequate relationships with our physicians is not wholly within our control; pressures on physicians' time, in particular those created by the demands of Health Maintenance Organizations (HMOs), compound the difficulty.[37] Among the concerns conscientious doctors have is that when they work under the aegis of HMOs they typically are restricted in the amount of time they can spend with patients.[38] Everyone knows that good communication takes time.

In fact, *time* may be at the core of the best sort of relationship—both the time for discussion during appointments and the time over an extended period that allows doctors and patients to become acquainted with and understand each other. The length of time Diane had been a patient of Timothy Quill's, and the months over which they worked out together how to achieve for her the best possible kind of death under unfortunate circumstances, is a good example of what is needed.[39]

There is no substitute for discussions between doctors and patients about a wide variety of matters beyond the obvious ones of what therapeutic measures are to be taken in a particular clinical situation. The truth

of this is even stronger when a patient is facing death. I have already alluded to many of the kinds of questions that need to be addressed: At
what point in the dying process is further medical treatment futile? How
is "futility" to be defined? Which medical interventions count as "ordinary" and which as "extraordinary"? Does a physician's role end when
cure is no longer possible, or is comfort care part of a physician's responsibility? And, critically and fundamentally, how does the physician interpret and understand "comfort care"? In a piece directed chiefly at
physicians, Megan McAndrew Cooper wrote (in the aftermath of her
husband's death) that it "should hurt to lose a patient for whom you have
tried so hard; if it doesn't, you are missing something that a doctor ought
to have. So at the end of our lives, when there is nothing else that you *can*
give, give us this: an acknowledgment of your own loss."[40] More doctors
need to learn to do this, more of the time.

Patients also need to talk with their physicians about the level of confidence that is appropriate in a physician's prognosis of remaining life.[41] It
would be helpful to doctors (and would improve doctor-patient dialogues)
if more patients realized that medical knowledge is inherently uncertain
and were able to discuss the implications of this phenomenon with their
physicians. Ideally, of course, such discussions would begin long before
a patient is dying. For example, does your doctor view the artificial con-
tinuation of nutrition and hydration as "medical treatment" and therefore
something you have a right to refuse? Or does your doctor believe feeding is in a special category (because there is a "psychological contiguity
between feeding and loving"[42])? If so, are struggles likely to be provoked
by your refusal to eat? Clearly, more is at issue than extended dialogue.
Social, ethical, and spiritual concerns all come into play—if we permit
them to.[43]

Knowing what position one's physician typically takes on end-of-life
care is not enough, by itself, of course. We need to explore which options
are truly open to us, and—in cooperation with our physicians—to come
to an understanding about what constitutes a legitimate continuum of care
at the end of life. Does a doctor's care at the end of a dying patient's life
stop with "comfort care"? Or is there a possible extension beyond what
that has come to mean, so that having a physician "ease the passage" (help
an ebbing life end sooner rather than later) could be the best way to render "comfort"—and "comfort *care*"? Those who feel most strongly about
autonomy and self-determination are likely to think that an unwillingness
to help them in this manner, which they conceive to be their right, is itself a failure to offer comfort.

One problem is that the phrase "comfort care" sometimes seems to have
been co-opted by the Hospice movement. (That it by no means does or
should belong uniquely to Hospice will become clear in the Profile of
Joanne Lynn that follows.) The phrase has begun to sound like a code for

something like "the way Hospice patients are cared for when curing them is no longer possible." As far as it goes, that is fine, and comfort care is indeed a fine thing. But a crucial part of the whole idea of "comfort care" has got to be the imaginative implementation of whatever will make patients more comfortable. In turn, that may well mean having the doctor take steps beyond simply eliminating or reducing pain, particularly when the only way to achieve that is to sedate the patient into mental oblivion ("terminal sedation," is the polite medical expression). That there is more than one way to understand the limits of "comfort care" could not be made clearer than by juxtaposing observations made by two of the persons profiled above, Cicely Saunders and Timothy Quill. In an editorial I quoted earlier, Saunders says: "Whatever our views on euthanasia, it surely cannot and should not be introduced as a logical part or extension of palliative care."[44] Bearing in mind that Saunders uses "euthanasia" to cover many things, including what physicians like Timothy Quill call "assisted dying," the divide between the two of them looms large and deep. Quill, it will be recalled, says this: "You definitely want [end of life care] on a continuum. The worst thing is having the doctor walk away. . . . I know when I am dying, I sure want a partner—a family member, of course, but also a medical partner if at all possible."

I think "comfort care" has real meaning for most people beyond the way it is restrictively used within the confines of the Hospice philosophy. It means not just keeping people comfortable so they can "live fully until they die," when cure is no longer possible; it means caring all the way through the process of dying itself for those who are ready for the end of life. I see no reason why "comfort" cannot also include, in extremis, what surgeon Francis D. Moore said was part of his credo: "[A]ssisting people to leave the dwelling place of their body when it is no longer habitable is becoming an obligation of the medical profession."[45]

Cicely Saunders is not the only one who would not share my sympathy with Moore's position.[46] But until "more sensible and representative policies are developed," Quill urges, "the only way to protect one's future is to develop a personal philosophy about one's own wishes . . . and then express it formally in an advance directive."[47] Even so, "obligation" is perhaps an unfortunate word for Moore to have used. As things currently stand, no doctor can be legally *required* to help bring a life to an end. Still, that does not mean it is inappropriate either for patients to ask their physicians to assume the obligation Moore recommends or for physicians to be willing to do so.

Part of the reason for urging that doctor-patient dialogue be initiated more earnestly and often is that it is one way to find out whether your physician is so adamantly opposed to the assistance you want in dying that there is no room for further discussion. Some doctors are completely opposed to performing euthanasia or doing anything that fits their definition of hastening death. We need to know whether this is the position our doctors take; if it is, and if that is not a position with which we are comfortable, we need to decide what to do about it. Are we content (for ourselves or others) with a situation that has some people dying not in the way they themselves want to, but in ways approved by others?[48] A letter to the editor by Cicely Saunders is an example of what gives rise to the concern that this could happen. Where good palliative care "is unavailable, or even unavailing, the few who might still find an 'enforced life' intolerable must call on our understanding and compassion," she says.[49] "Just trust us" is what it sounds like. We should perhaps not be surprised that some supporters of Hemlock find "the hospice movement's denial of choice to be totalitarian."[50]

If we think "compassion" may be what dying patients seek above all, we surely have to leave room for the patient's own definition of compassion. Some doctors' experiences lead them to believe that the "right to die" is not "a burning issue with most people"; despite caring for many dying patients they have had very few (perhaps even none) ask for help in ending their lives.[51] But it does not follow that all doctors and patients will have the same experiences. Furthermore, no *un*willing health-care provider is going to be required to assist a patient in dying, because even if there is a right to die it is not a general claim-right against any (let alone every) provider of health-care services. As we have seen, my right to die cannot entail a duty for anyone else to come forward and end my life for me. Yet doctors who are not willing providers must nonetheless be willing in one respect, namely, willing to suggest other more sympathetic physicians. Doctors need to be tolerant not only in general of the different cultures out of which their patients come, but also very specifically of the different standards according to which autonomous individuals are free to act. Doctors and patients both need to work—together—on improving end-of-life care.

PROFILE: JOANNE LYNN[52]

Trying to arrange a time to meet with Joanne Lynn turned out to be a little like throwing additional balls to a juggler; at first I couldn't seem to get the balls quite within her range, though it was clear she was more than prepared to catch them. Actually, it was telephone tag we were playing, followed by a comedy of errors with schedules that refused to mesh. She was in Boston when I was in Washington, and vice versa; I had to turn down two different invitations to dinner at her home because my arrival in D.C. didn't quite fit with dinners she had already arranged. And so it went; I almost gave up. But curiosity about this busy woman whose career is marked by an unusual number of twists and turns, combined with

my high regard for several elderly doctors who had spoken enthusiasti-
cally about Lynn's efforts on behalf of the dying, made me persist. In the
end I was very glad I did, despite several odd features of the visit.

The day arrived at last, when I was in Washington and she was free—
in a manner of speaking. If I would take a cab to her home in McLean,
Virginia, we could talk over a late lunch. Fine, I said. And so I set off.

When it becomes clear I will arrive well ahead of the appointed time, I
dismiss the cab so I can walk the rest of the way—and the strangeness of
my visit begins. Here I am, wandering along a road in near-rural McLean,
trying to avoid cars (no sidewalk, of course) and trying to look as if I know
where I am going. My timing works out just about right, however, and I
arrive at precisely the appointed time. No one is home. I feel foolish, stuck
out in the country with no phone, no hope of a cab back to D.C., and no
sign of the person I have come to see.

I needn't have worried. Just as I am beginning to feel really awkward,
Dr. Lynn pulls into the driveway with her son in tow. *She* doesn't appear
to see any oddity in my standing there in the front yard waiting for her.
She welcomes me in as if we are neighbors about to have coffee together.
I can see this will be no formal interview.

Thus it comes about that my first opportunity to make a personal assessment of Joanne Lynn—doctor, medical administrator, public policy
advocate, teacher, lecturer—is in her roles as housewife and mother. The
son has not been well; her gentle concern over his welfare is palpable, and
she talks openly of it rather than trying to disguise or brush aside the need
to attend to him. Of course strictly it was irrelevant, but I realize later that
this melding of her family and professional responsibilities is a hallmark
of the way she does what she does. Casually dressed in a simple sweater-
and-skirt outfit, bustling about the kitchen, she could be a superannuated
graduate student, a newcomer to the study of death-and-dying. Instead,
though there is no outward hint of it, she is a distinguished expert not only
on how to offer high-quality care to the dying, but on topics such as
medical decision-making, the efficacy of medical intervention, and health-
care policy. She is in her late forties, I would guess; she is famous, smart,
hardworking, much in demand—and utterly unpretentious. I like this; I
begin to be amused by the circumstances of our meeting.

The house is in chaos; Lynn and her family have just moved in. She
shows me her teen-aged daughter's room (I don't remember why), evidence of a mother who is willing to grant children their space; it's a classic mess that makes me wonder how the girl gets safely in and out.
Throughout the downstairs of the house, there are boxes of family pos-
sessions not yet fully unpacked. Piles of laundry wait to be done. If my
house looked like that when a stranger came to visit, for whatever reason, I would be embarrassed. Joanne Lynn on the other hand shows not

a flicker of distress over the disarray, nor does she give any sign she thinks she needs to apologize or explain beyond the one or two sentences having to do with her son's health and the recent move.

Okay, I'm fine with this, I think, as I follow her into the kitchen. Lunch, it turns out, will be a cup of instant soup, which we carry into the formal dining room with its not-yet-lived-in look. This, too, is fine with me. I share news with Lynn about my aging doctor-friends in Hanover, New Hampshire (where she was recently on the Dartmouth Medical School faculty and a senior associate at Dartmouth's Center for the Evaluative Clinical Sciences). I report on my academic interests in doctor-patient relations and the relationship between doctors and their dying patients in particular. And she responds, answers questions, challenges with questions of her own. Throughout my visit, I have the distinct impression that Joanne Lynn is engaged simultaneously in half a dozen tasks of a wide variety, but that she never, ever, loses concentration or focus. This juggler doesn't drop any ball that is remotely within reach.

Some of what I know of Dr. Lynn comes from listening to the tape of a forum on physician-assisted suicide in which she participated. The forum, in the spring of 1992, was co-sponsored by Dartmouth's Institute for the Study of Applied and Professional Ethics and the Tucker Foundation; it was held at a retirement community (Kendal at Hanover), home to a number of my friends (those aging doctors). I was not present for the program but I was able to borrow the tape and talk to several people who were there; I also read an edited transcript of the forum.[53] This proves to have been a good introduction to Lynn's style, which is direct, outspoken, honest, self-revealing. What you see is what you get. It's also true of what you hear; there is no artifice. Just so on my visit to her home. Nothing of relevance, one feels, is hidden. Where ideas about how doctors should behave are concerned—particularly when it comes to caring for dying patients—it is always open season for Joanne Lynn. At least that is what she conveys to me, on tape and in person.

The blunt honesty, coupled with a skill I've noticed in her writing (capturing truths in compact and memorable phrases), is what I like best. Ideas and thoughts and considered opinions flow so fast and freely that I can't jot anything down as a precise quote. But her views are clear: Any putative "denial of death" is not nearly so significant as the fact that talk about death (especially one's own) is generally considered inappropriate for polite public discourse. What people call "decisions"—the actions taken at various points of demarcation along the way toward death—are in fact made without any of the usual trappings of true decision-making. Whom, she seems to be asking, do we think we are kidding?

We have to get used to the idea that there are "different trajectories of death," Lynn's way of saying that not everybody dies the same way. The segue into the need for us as a society to establish—get used to—a new category of patients is smooth. The real issue is how we are going to deal with the chronically (or long-term—don't pretend these are the same) life-impacted individuals who are not going to get better (for example, those with multiple sclerosis or Alzheimer's) but who are not "dying" or even, in common parlance, "terminally ill."

Joanne Lynn's experience as one of the co-principal investigators on the SUPPORT study—the results of which were published subsequent to my visit—seems to have turned her into more of a spokesperson for the (dying) elderly than ever. She is frequently called upon to interpret and explain how it could be that better communication between doctors and dying patients doesn't necessarily solve problems. In her introduction to Marilyn Webb's *The Good Death* (1997), while talking about what we could (and should) do to help "[f]amilies and nursing homes . . . learn how to make good on the promise of old age, even with illness and disability," she lays out this challenge: "We could do better. We could set about reshaping our social institutions so that the end of life is worthy and valid, comfortable and comforted. Some of what needs to be done lies in the realms of public policy and professional education—to change Medicare reimbursement formulas, to demand measurement of the quality of care, and to learn the new sets of skills for professional caregivers, for example."[54]

This focus on practical ways to make life easier for dying patients is typical of Lynn. Part of the reason she opposes physician-assisted dying is that she knows there is much more we could be doing for the dying besides pain palliation. She believes doing some of that much more would minimize the apparent need for the kind of "assistance" represented by physician-aid-in-dying, legalized or otherwise. "It is easier to get a hip replaced or to get ICU [Intensive Care Unit] care than it is to get a backrub and a bath—and that is crazy," she said during the Dartmouth forum. This epigrammatic way of focusing the problem is characteristic of the way she talks. (She has a knack for cutting to the chase. "It is easier to get open-heart surgery than Meals on Wheels," is another classic Lynn line.[55])

Opposed though Lynn is to adding physician-assisted suicide to the doctor's armamentarium, she sees much in the current state of affairs that is unacceptable. "I do think there are a lot of rituals in medicine that are very dysfunctional, and I'm not defending the way we currently manage dying," she has said. "Dying is commonly lonely and it is commonly a source of bankruptcy. The way we fail to support people with serious chronic diseases is a national scandal. We are the only civilized Western nation that has no program of community support for people who are unable to care for themselves."[56]

Furthermore, she insists, one way to improve the care of the dying is to "attend to our language"; there is "no term that is more vacuous and misleading than 'the terminally ill.' The difference between being mortal and being terminally ill is a very hard line to find. The arrogance of establishing a category of 'other' that is called 'terminally ill' is a way of distancing ourselves from the fact that we're all dying."[57]

Though someone who did not know Lynn might think there was a kind of "Take *that!*" quality to much of what she writes and says, my visit with her tells me otherwise. When I read the paper in which that last set of remarks appeared a year or so after my visit, I could virtually hear her voice again. Blunt and plainspoken perhaps, yes, but there is nothing coarse or unkind in her manner. It's just that there is a job to be done, and she sees herself in a position to do it. So this is how it is, she seems to be saying, and this is what we are going to do about it. Part of the "what we are going to do about it" is found in the Center to Improve Care of the Dying that she now heads at George Washington University.

Another part is in the organization she founded shortly after returning to Washington from Dartmouth, the Americans for Better Care of the Dying (ABCD) that I mentioned in Chapter 2. A four-page flyer put out by ABCD in mid-2001 makes manifest the sweeping reforms Lynn and her organization have in mind. It opens with "A Vision of a Better System," the goals of ABCD, and then has three "Action Guide" pages directed at four constituencies: clinicians, benefits managers and purchasers, citizens, and policymakers.

Given Lynn's opposition to physician-assisted suicide and her years of experience as a Hospice medical director, it is perhaps surprising to hear her also saying, again bluntly, that "Hospice is not the answer." She comes to that conclusion not because Hospice is ineffective or a bad idea, but because it does not, and cannot, serve everyone. Palliative care, too, needs to be provided "much more sensibly and comprehensively. I do not want to see us 'stop treatment and switch to palliative care.' I want palliative care all the time."[58] So there. She is, above all, an advocate for the ill and the dying. "When people talk about dying," she points out, "they tend to mean the last day. But [dying] is about how to live well despite the fact that you have a condition that will end up taking your life."[59]

I like this no-nonsense practical approach to what too often remains an esoteric and philosophical question of rights and moral legitimacy and integrity of the profession. After lunch, Lynn gives me a ride to the Metro station. We disagree on some important issues, but I don't see how anyone could be working harder than she is to make this dying business less difficult. "Using what we already know to help the dying must be a priority," she says.[60] And Joanne Lynn is doing just that. I see in her a real hope for the future; her reasons for arguing that Hospice is not the whole answer leave open the possibility of tolerance for other approaches. Maybe, even, Hemlock; I don't know. But I am struck by how quickly I am drawn in by her energy. I respect her capacity to do that, just as I cannot fail to respect her.

NOTES

1. Simon Dach (my translation), from *"Wie? ist es denn night gnug, einmal sterben wollen?"* ("What? Is it not enough, just to want to die?"), in Walther Ziesemer, ed., *Gedichte,* 4 vols., (Halle/Salle: Max Niemeyer Verlag, 1936): vol. 1, 203–04.

2. Hastings Center, *Guidelines on the Termination of Life-Sustaining Treatment and the Care of the Dying* (Bloomington: Indiana University Press, 1987).

3. Reinhard Priester and Robert Koepp, eds., *Termination of Treatment of Adults* (Center for Biomedical Ethics, University of Minnesota, 1993), p. 1. The ground-breaking attempt to establish a check list of principles for medical decision-making is in Tom L. Beauchamp and James F. Childress, eds., *Principles of Biomedical Ethics* (New York: Oxford University Press, 1979).

4. Hastings Center, *Guidelines,* pp. 18–19; the terms in parentheses are the ones used in Priester and Koepp, eds., *Termination of Treatment,* p. 1.

5. The President's Commission for the Study of Ethical Problems in Medicine and Biomedical and Behavioral Research, *Deciding to Forego Life-Sustaining Treatment* (Mar. 1983), p. 132 (in Priester and Koepp, eds., *Termination of Treatment,* p. 27) uses this language, as do Priester and Koepp themselves, p. 1.

6. Elizabeth L. Beardsley, "Privacy: Autonomy and Selective Disclosure," in J. Roland Pennock and John W. Chapman, eds., *Privacy, NOMOS XIII* (New York: Atherton Press, 1971), p. 59.

7. Mark Siegler, "Critical Illness: The Limits of Autonomy," *HCR* 7, no. 5 (Oct. 1977): 12–15.

8. Bruce L. Miller, "Autonomy and the Refusal of Lifesaving Treatment," *HCR* 11, no. 4 (Aug. 1981): 24–25.

9. David A. Asch, John Hansen-Flaschen, and Paul N. Lanken, "Decisions to Limit or Continue Life-sustaining Treatment by Critical Care Physicians in the United States: Conflicts Between Physicians' Practices and Patients' Wishes," *Am. Jrnl. of Resp. and Crit. Care Med.* 151 (1995): 288.

10. Lawrence J. Schneiderman, Nancy S. Jecker, and Albert R. Jonsen, "Medical Futility: Its Meaning and Ethical Implications," *Ann. of Int. Med.* 112, no. 12 (15 June 1990): 953.

11. Schneiderman, Jecker, and Jonsen, "Medical Futility," *Ann. of Int. Med.:* 953.

12. Donald J. Murphy, "Do-Not-Resuscitate Orders: Time for Reappraisal in Long-term–Care Institutions," *JAMA* 260, no. 14 (14 Oct. 1988): 2100.

13. Stuart J. Youngner, "Who Defines Futility?" *JAMA* 260, no. 14 (14 Oct. 1988): 2095.

14. See the President's Commission, *Deciding to Forego,* p. 132 (in Priester and Koepp, eds., *Termination of Treatment,* p. 27).

15. Charles Baron, "On Taking Substituted Judgment Seriously," *HCR* 20, no. 5 (Sept.-Oct. 1990): 8.

16. In fact, "integrity of the profession" is sometimes omitted and replaced with "non-maleficence," probably on the ground that professional integrity is precisely what "beneficence" and "non-maleficence" taken together mean. For example, four of the key chapters in Beauchamp and Childress, eds., *Principles of Biomedical Ethics,* are titled "The Principle of Autonomy," "The Principle of Non-maleficence," "The Principle of Beneficence," and "The Principle of Justice." There

is no "Principle of the Integrity of the Profession" (though one chapter is called "The Professional and Patient Relationship").

17. Timothy E. Quill, *Death and Dignity: Making Choices and Taking Charge* (New York: Norton, 1993), p. 106.

18. Marcia Angell, "Medicine: The Endangered Patient-Centered Ethic," *HCR* 17, no. 1 (Feb. 1987): Special Supplement, 12.

19. Norman Daniels, *Just Health Care* (Cambridge: Cambridge University Press, 1985). I am much indebted to this book, in general, for what follows in my text.

20. John Rawls, "Justice as Fairness," *Phil. Rev.* 67, no. 2 (Apr. 1958): 164–94. Rawls later expanded his ideas first in his major treatise, *A Theory of Justice* (Cambridge, Mass.: Harvard University Press, 1971), and more recently in (Erin Kelly, ed.) *Justice as Fairness: A Restatement* (Cambridge, Mass.: Harvard University Press, 2001).

21. Rawls, *Theory,* p. 83, and Daniels, *Just Health Care,* p. 33. Daniels defines "Normal Opportunity Range" in a species-typical manner; he also accepts Rawls's distinction between a *formal* or merely legal requirement of equality of opportunity and a truly "fair equality of opportunity."

22. See Humphry's homepage on the Web at *http://www.FinalExit.org/dhumphry.*

23. Reinhard Priester and Robert Koepp, eds., *Withholding or Withdrawing Artificial Nutrition and Hydration* (Center for Biomedical Ethics, University of Minnesota, 1993), p. 11n28.

24. Thomas J. Prendergast, "Finding meaning," *Dartmouth Med.* (Winter 1999): 31.

25. Timothy Quill, personal communication.

26. Such cases come up with distressing frequency. A classic is that of Diane Pretty in England, who—severely incapacitated by (and dying of, but not deemed "terminally ill" from) motor neuron disease, caused a stir in mid-2001 by going public with her fight to be allowed to have a medically assisted death at a time of her own choosing. See Tracy McVeigh, "'I just want to choose how I die. It's my life,'" *The [London] Observer* (24 June 2001): 3; also Len Doyal and Lesley Doyal, "Why euthanasia and physician assisted suicide should be legalised," *BMJ* 323 (10 Nov. 2001): 1079–80. Late in November 2001, Pretty lost her appeal to the House of Lords. Jill Lawless, "British court denies patient right to die with spouse's help," *BG* (30 Nov. 2001): A18.

27. Tom L. Beauchamp and Seymour Perlin, eds., *Ethical Issues in Death and Dying* (Englewood Cliffs, N.J.: Prentice-Hall, 1978), pp. 217–18.

28. Dan W. Brock, *Life and Death: Philosophical Essays in Biomedical Ethics* (Cambridge: Cambridge University Press, 1993), p. 409.

29. Abraham Kaplan, "Social Ethics and the Sanctity of Life: A Summary," in Daniel H. Labby, ed., *Life or Death: Ethics and Options* (Seattle: University of Washington Press, 1968), p. 153.

30. Rawls, *Theory,* pp. 20, 49. In contrast to Rawls, Judith Thomson insists that "some moral judgments are plausibly viewed as necessary truths and hence not open to revision." Judith Jarvis Thomson, *The Realm of Rights* (Cambridge, Mass.: Harvard University Press, 1990), p. 32n20.

31. I have based my formulation of the principles mainly on Beauchamp and Perlin, eds., *Ethical Issues;* Vincent Mor, David S. Greer, and Robert Kastenbaum, eds., *The Hospice Experiment* (Baltimore: Johns Hopkins University Press, 1988);

Anne Munley, *The Hospice Alternative: A New Context for Death and Dying* (New York: Basic Books, 1983); and Louis P. Pojman, ed., *Life and Death: A Reader in Moral Problems* (Boston: Jones & Bartlett, 1993).

32. Quill, *Death and Dignity*, p. 105.

33. Richard W. Momeyer, *Confronting Death* (Bloomington: Indiana University Press, 1988), p. 14.

34. Daniel C. Maguire, *Death by Choice* (New York: Schocken Books, 1975), p. 131.

35. Constance E. Putnam, "Who talks? Who listens? Who decides? Doctors and patients in discourse," in Frans H. van Eemeren, Rob Grootendorst, J. Anthony Blair, and Charles A. Willard, eds., 4 vols., *Proceedings of the Third ISSA Conference on Argumentation* (Amsterdam: Sic Sat, 1995), vol. 4, p. 419. Too many of those exploring shared decision-making in the contemporary world of medicine are, I believe, unduly optimistic about improvements to date. See, e.g., Ezekiel J. Emanuel and Linda L. Emanuel, "Four Models of the Physician-Patient Relationship," *JAMA* 267, no. 16 (22/29 Apr. 1992): 2221–26; and Mark Siegler, "The Progression of Medicine: From Physician Paternalism to Patient Autonomy to Bureaucratic Parsimony," *Arch. of Int. Med.* 145 (Apr. 1985): 713–15. But see also Stephen G. Post, "Beyond Adversity: Physician and Patient as Friends?" *Jrnl. of Med. Humanities* 15, no. 1 (Spring 1994): 23–29; Howard Waitzkin, *The Politics of Medical Encounters: How Patients and Doctors Deal with Social Problems* (New Haven, Conn.: Yale University Press, 1991), esp. pp. 27–48 and 259–77; and Vilhjálmur Árnason, "Towards Authentic Conversations: Authenticity in the Patient-Professional Relationship," *Theoretical Med.* 15 (1994): 227–42.

36. William A. Knaus and Joanne Lynn, et al. (SUPPORT Principal Investigators), "A Controlled Trial to Improve Care for Seriously Ill Hospitalized Patients: The Study to Understand Prognoses and Preferences for Outcomes and Risks of Treatments (SUPPORT)," *JAMA* 274, no. 20 (22–29 Nov. 1995): 1591–98. See also the accompanying editorial: Bernard Lo, "Improving Care Near the End of Life: Why Is It So Hard?" *JAMA* 274, no. 20 (22–29 Nov. 1995): 1634–36.

37. See, e.g., Richard A. Knox, "The rush is on—in doctors' offices," *BG* (2 Mar. 1996): 1; but see also a doctor arguing that managed care actually improves the way time is spent, in Robert A. Witzburg (letter to the editor), "Age-old question: Are doctors too rushed?" *BG* (11 Mar. 1996): 10.

38. See, e.g., Leonard Laster, "Let the patient beware," *BG* (5 Nov. 1995): 81, 85.

39. See Timothy E. Quill, "Death and Dignity: A Case of Individualized Decision Making," *NEJM* 324, no. 10 (7 Mar. 1991): 691–94.

40. Megan McAndrew Cooper, "Acknowledgment of loss," in *Dartmouth Med.* (Winter 1999): 30.

41. Nicholas Christakis, a hospice doctor and associate professor of sociology and medicine at the University of Chicago, has done research on just this issue: How well doctors predict their patients' outcomes and how well they do "in helping dying patients spend their remaining time without pain and among their family members." For an interview with Christakis, see Gina Kolata, "A Doctor With a Cause: 'What's My Prognosis?'" *NYT* (28 Nov. 2000): D7.

42. Joanne Lynn and James F. Childress, "Must Patients Always Be Given Food and Water?" in Joanne Lynn, ed., *By No Extraordinary Means* (Bloomington: Indiana University Press, 1986), p. 48.

43. See, e.g., Clive Seale, "Social and ethical aspects of euthanasia: a review," *Progress in Palliative Care* 5, no. 4 (1997): 141–46.

44. Cicely Saunders, "Voluntary euthanasia," *Palliative Med.* 6 (1992): 1.

45. Francis D. Moore, "Prolonging Life, Permitting Life to End," *Harvard Mag.* 97, no. 6 (July-Aug. 1995): 47.

46. See, e.g., five expressions of a range of reactions to his article in the letters column of the magazine's next issue, under the rubric "Life . . . and Death's Dominion," *Harvard Mag.* 98, no. 1 (Sept.-Oct. 1995): 4–5.

47. Quill, *Death and Dignity*, p. 188.

48. See Ronald Dworkin, *Life's Dominion: An Argument About Abortion, Euthanasia, and Individual Freedom* (New York: Knopf, 1993), p. 217, for his take on this.

49. Cicely Saunders (letter to the editor), "Enforced death: enforced life," *Jrnl. of Med. Ethics* 18, no. 1 (Mar. 1992): 48.

50. Ludovic Kennedy, *Euthanasia: The Good Death* (London: Chatto & Windus, 1990), p. 30, attributing this view to physician Colin Brewer.

51. Lynn Sheffey, personal communication.

52. Based on a visit to Lynn's home in McLean, Virginia, on March 30, 1996.

53. [Forum,] "Should Doctors Hasten Death?" *Dartmouth Med.* (Fall 1992): 34–41, 64.

54. Joanne Lynn, "Introduction," in Marilyn Webb, *The Good Death: The New American Search to Reshape the End of Life* (New York: Bantam Books, 1997), p. xviii.

55. Joanne Lynn, "Caring for Those Who Die in Old Age," in Howard M. Spiro, Mary G. McCrea Curnen, and Lee Palmer Wandel, eds., *Facing Death: Where Culture, Religion, and Medicine Meet* (New Haven, Conn.: Yale University Press, 1996), p. 99.

56. [Forum,] "Should Doctors Hasten Death?" *Dartmouth Med.*: 37.

57. Lynn, "Caring for Those Who Die," p. 98.

58. Lynn, "Caring for Those Who Die," pp. 98–99.

59. Joanne Lynn, quoted in Kate Muir, "Living well at the end of life," *The [London] Times* (9 June 1999): 19.

60. Lynn, "Caring for Those Who Die," p. 99.

6

Death Matters

Death freely chosen is not the worst possible death.
—Simone de Beauvoir[1]

Tell them I've had a wonderful life.
—Ludwig Wittgenstein[2]

In my opening chapter, I raised a pair of questions to get us started: How does one begin thinking critically and systematically about the elusive, difficult, and anxiety-inducing question of how to face death? What are the implications of what we *think* we think about the matter? At the end of that chapter, I posed another, compound, question: To what extent do Hospice and Hemlock, separately or together, adequately reflect values held to be central in contemporary American society—and do these movements (again, separately or together) give adequate room for physicians to exercise the kind of heroic compassion toward the dying that such persons seem concerned to receive? Posed alternatively: How does one go about figuring out what it is appropriate for dying patients to expect by way of help from their physicians, and can either Hospice or Hemlock alone provide that?

In the succeeding chapters, we have massaged in a variety of ways these questions as well as more personal ones implicit in the initial questions. We have uncovered what I hope are either answers or ways of finding out what the answers might be on the most personal level. The time has now come to look at the consequences for society as a whole. I will address this constellation of issues before attempting to state where my reflections on Hospice, Hemlock, and the end of life lead when compassion for the dying person is the first priority.

COMMON GROUND, COMPROMISES, AND CONCLUSIONS

Can putting principles into practice and unpacking arguments, as we did in the previous chapter, point us in the direction of a workable compromise between Hospice and Hemlock? Does a better understanding of the arguments behind the positions increase the likelihood of reaching agreements on where limits should be set for individuals within the context of the larger community? If we re-examine more closely what appears to be the common ground on which Hospice and Hemlock stand, we see that although both favor pain control and stress the importance of palliative care, even there differences exist. And these differences in turn shed light on the other, more sharply drawn disagreements between the movements.

Let's look first at the attitude toward pain control. The insistence that no one should have to die alone or in pain—central to Hospice philosophy—is far more remarkable than one might first think. To a distressing extent, the dying process in contemporary society is for many people riddled with pain. When the business of dying drags on for a long time, much of that time is also often spent alone.

The reasons for this are not far to seek. With something like 75 percent of deaths in the United States taking place in medical facilities of one sort or another,[3] the circle of friends and family members once typically gathered around the dying person has largely disappeared. That speaks to the issue of dying alone; less easily understood is why pain is so often a major feature of the landscape for those who are dying. It has been asserted that the "arsenal of weapons" available to doctors to ease pain in the dying process is too little used, "due largely to the ignorance of many physicians."[4] One might suppose (or hope) that dying in a hospital would make pain medications readily accessible. But while access to medication may indeed be easier in medical institutions, in principle, modern practice at least in the United States continues to downplay the extent to which patients may need palliation. Sometimes the justification lies in a failure to understand pain or a lack of knowledge about ways to alleviate it; sometimes it seems rather to be an outgrowth of a defensive approach to the practice of medicine that emerges from a fear of malpractice suits. Too much in the way of analgesics might kill the patient, the fear goes; better to under-medicate and not run the risk. Cynics incline toward the view that those who reason this way have a "So what if, in the meantime, the patient suffers?" attitude. More sympathetic observers accept as a principle that some pain is probably unavoidable and that those who err on the side of caution are not to be faulted. Either way, pain relief rarely seems to be the top priority for those in charge of medical care.

But such common ground as Hospice and Hemlock share on the issue of pain turns muddy once pain has been successfully alleviated. For Hospice, palliation—though an important goal—is not necessarily seen as an end in itself. Rather, it is (perhaps primarily) a means of making it possible for patients to live life fully until the end. If that is to happen, patients must be freed as much as possible from pain and other unwanted distractions and sources of distress. For many clinicians within the Hospice movement, this period when life is ebbing but pain has been (largely) controlled is first and foremost a period for spiritual growth. It is a time for taking care of "unfinished business" with God or in interpersonal relations, or for generally coming to terms with the way one's life has unfolded.

For those on the Hemlock side, palliation comes closer to being an end in itself. Being as free from pain as one can reasonably be made is no more than what any rational individual would want (though those who choose not to have their pain alleviated of course have the right to dispense with palliation). But there is another, far more important, issue within Hemlock. Even when pain has been satisfactorily dealt with, spiritual growth or doing the "work" of dying is generally not the main consideration. Rather, most Hemlock supporters hold a firm conviction that one has a right to dispose of one's own affairs—including choosing to end one's life; autonomy is the key value.

Many Hospice supporters also talk about how each death is individual and how people have choices, to be sure, but "choice" in Hospice circles is rarely so inclusively understood as in Hemlock circles. Dr. Ira Byock (a prominent but at times controversial figure in the Hospice world[5]) tells numerous stories in his book of a few years ago in part to demonstrate that "the actual experience of dying is not captured by a purely medical perspective that sees only problems." Dying, he says, is a "profoundly personal experience."[6] Still, Hospice advocates are likely to share a kind of certainty about what that profoundly personal, final journey should look like. Hemlock supporters, on the other hand, maintain that no one can know for someone else what the end should look like and that no one should have the right to impose on another his or her conception of what is appropriate. There are physicians, too, who lose patience over what they see as the self-importance of Hospice people: "They view themselves as the champions on white horses riding in to save the day. The hospice approach often is too rigid, expecting—even demanding—that death be this fantastic event when all relationships are mended and life is neatly wrapped up," one physician complained to a reporter.[7] Here lies the central element of the disagreement.

This takes us directly back to the second pairing of principles in the previous chapter: Hospice P_2 ("Affirming life means doing nothing to prolong or delay the dying process; human dignity is maintained by living life fully to the end.") and Hemlock P_4 ("An individual's life is his or her own—and only the individual in question can know when that life has reached its tolerable limits, when the maintenance of personal dignity permits making a choice in favor of death."). In this clash of principles, Hospice and Hemlock do not merely superficially disagree; they actually diverge. For Hospice, getting rid of pain is important above all as a step toward something else of greater importance. For Hemlock, alleviation of pain is also a good, but one that is often almost incidental to the real point—the autonomous person's freedom of choice and right to self-determination. Thus, although Hemlock proponents welcome (actively seek and applaud) the removal of pain, they will not be likely to change their minds about who should be making the end-of-life decisions. In other words, their position would be this: Take away my pain (thank you very much), but I still want to make my own decisions about the end of my own life. Indeed, *I have a right* to do so. If others make these decisions, they will be acting in a paternalistic manner that has now fallen largely into disrepute. The crux of the dispute is over rights and autonomy.[8]

More remains to be said about how compromises might be reached with respect to such a fundamental disagreement. But we can already see the way the scales probably need to be tipped. At first blush, it might seem that the best solution for a whole society is likely to lie in principles that apply generally. That is precisely what the Hospice principles are intended to do. However, a society is not normally homogeneous in all respects. Most especially, when one thinks of the collectivity known as "human beings," the range and variety within the group are so enormous that it is imperative to limit the number of universal claims and to construe them very narrowly. Supporters of Hospice P_1 ("Dying is a natural life-cycle process that ought not necessarily to include suffering, the fear of suffering, or loneliness; no one who does not choose to should have to die alone or in pain.") and Hospice P_2 ("Affirming life means doing nothing to prolong or delay the dying process; human dignity is maintained by living life fully to the end.") frequently do truly believe that their position is one that should be followed by all. The problem lies in the fact that one of the premises establishing Hospice P_2, in particular, with its (largely Christian) theological basis, is sectarian. By definition, then, it is a principle with which many are bound to disagree. Furthermore, it is a principle in absolute and direct conflict with the premise under Hemlock P_4 that places responsibility for making the "right" decision squarely on the individual.

What is needed is a way to respect the differences that exist between and among individuals within the society (the larger group) to which those individuals belong. The fundamental question on which all controversy about the right to die rests, Ronald Dworkin has pointed out, is this: "Does a decent government attempt to dictate to its citizens what intrinsic values they will recognize, and why, and how?"[9] His implied answer is negative. If a "decent government" should not attempt to dictate on such points, how much less should any single group—even such a broadly conceived group as that represented by the Hospice movement—determine for others what they should believe and do.

Of course in principle no one is coerced into entering hospice care. Yet palliative care of the sort Hospice has made into a specialty is still most often available under the auspices of officially affiliated Hospice units. Furthermore, with a government-supported Hospice benefit in place, the choice *not* to become a Hospice patient may be bought at a steep price.[10] A competent adult individual's right to decide for him- or herself when there is no harm to others should be paramount, but some of that may get lost in a Hospice environment. Sidney Wanzer makes the point succinctly, stressing the importance of making sure end-of-life treatment is carried out at the simplest level possible. A patient who remains at home, for example, is likely to retain far more control than one who is confined in a hospital.[11]

In fact, in a liberal democratic society, it is difficult to see how differences among persons and peoples can be respected without a strong underlying regard for individual rights. Diversity is a fact of life in the modern world, cyberspace and international mobility notwithstanding. Organizing an entire society on sectarian principles will not work without severe repression of the rights of those who are not part of the dominant sect. The solution, it seems to me, must be to structure the principles according to which society operates in such a way that non-sectarian principles override sectarian principles—by assuring that room is provided for freedom of choice.[12]

In other words, *permitting* should trump *prohibiting*. If you do not approve of something I choose to do, you certainly have a right to try to dissuade me (rationally, by exercising your right to free speech, for example). But if I am not persuaded, you may not prohibit me from doing what I choose to do if it does not directly infringe the rights of anyone else. Neither may I stand in the way of your ability to choose not to do whatever it is you find offensive in my action. We put ourselves at risk by forgetting or ignoring these points. The problem, of course, is that sectarian beliefs may include values that declare some activities to be wrong under all circumstances for all people. Murder and suicide are among the favorites (and in this context the most relevant) examples. Those who believe suicide and murder are universally wrong, and that ending one's own life or getting assistance from a physician to bring life to an end is a form of suicide or murder, will have difficulty seeing why society should allow such actions under any circumstances.

The main issue, to repeat, is one of *who should have control over whom.* Is ultimate control to be in the hands of sectarian groups to which only a fraction of the society belongs? Or should it be in the hands of society as a whole (represented by the government)? If the latter, should that social control reflect what is seen as best from the point of view of the medical establishment or of some other particular institution? (This can easily turn sectarian.) Or should control rest with the individual? Daniel Callahan is quick to deride our desire to control everything, including death—a recurring theme in his *Troubled Dream of Life* (1993)[13]—and he uses the inappropriateness of this drive to control as an argument against physician-aid-in-dying. But Callahan and other proponents of Hospice seem not to notice that they are promoting what at times amounts to the exercise of a different kind of control when they insist that physician-aid-in-dying is *not* appropriate. They want death to take place in the way *they* deem acceptable, which means without any acts (of commission or omission) that will intentionally hasten the time of death.

Peter Steinfels, writing in the *New York Times* (hence for a very wide audience), said that for (most?) "Americans, the great solvent of ethical dilemmas is individual, private choice." But he went on to point out that some of the complications currently "rippling throughout the health care system show how inescapably social even such an ostensibly private choice can be."[14] Our challenge, both individually and as a society, is to keep the social from being controlled by the sectarian.

The values around issues of life and death that come most sharply into conflict with each other in a diverse society are often cast in terms of the "sanctity of life," and these are powerful values. Troublingly, however, the sanctity of life is often made to appear to stand in opposition to the right to self-determination. In other words, those who talk most vociferously about the sanctity of life tend to make it sound as if those who are concerned with self-determination are *not* interested in (or do not believe in) the sanctity of life. This is unlikely to be true. Even though it is often explicitly asserted that "Hospice affirms life" (a nice way to capture the rhetorical high ground, as I pointed out earlier), it does not follow that Hemlock somehow neglects to affirm, or *dis*affirms, life. Furthermore, as Ronald Dworkin has noted, there is more than one way to show the respect for human life that is inherent in the idea of the sanctity of life. Dworkin reminds us that "the instinct that deliberate death is a savage insult to the intrinsic value of life" is "central to many religious traditions." And yet, he urges his readers to remember, the sanctity of life is "both more complex, and more open to different and competing interpretations, than its religious use sometimes acknowledges."[15] Keeping powerful values like self-determination or autonomy and the sanctity of life from fatally clashing with each other is not easy. A critical first step is to understand that opposition to suicide, euthanasia, and physician-aid-in-dying may well rest on a misapprehension about the sanctity of life. Summing up, Dworkin puts this sensitive issue as follows:

[T]he question posed by euthanasia is not whether the sanctity of life should yield to some other value, like humanity or compassion, but how life's sanctity should be understood and respected. The great moral issues of abortion and euthanasia, which bracket life in earnest, have a similar structure. Each involves decisions not just about the rights and interests of particular people, but about the intrinsic, cosmic importance of human life itself. In each case, opinions divide not because some people have contempt for values that others cherish, but, on the contrary, because the values in question are at the center of everyone's lives, and no one can treat them as trivial enough to accept other people's orders about what they mean. Making someone die in a way that others approve, but he believes a horrifying contradiction of his life, is a devastating, odious form of tyranny.[16]

I would argue, with Dworkin, that "sanctity of life" arguments can and do work as much or more in favor of allowing euthanasia as against it. As a consequence, I wish also to suggest, it has to be the case that "Hospice" and "Hemlock" are not necessarily or inherently in opposition. Adherents of both groups believe in the sanctity of life; adherents of both groups seek a better life as well as a better death for the dying. Careful arguments will show that despite differences, there is, indeed, common ground we can traverse together.

CONSEQUENCES AND IMPLICATIONS FOR SOCIETY

What, then, would be the likely consequences for society if patients were more free to ask for physician-aid-in-dying? Surely there is no danger in arranging things so that patients are free to *ask*. Granting freedom to make a request is a long way from saying that the request must be fulfilled. Furthermore, free and open discussion is the only way that this topic of life-and-death importance can be brought "over ground, instead of underground," as Timothy Quill puts it.

Among the most distressing features of the current situation (one that has prevailed for some time, actually) is that even when patients do ask, doctors either don't listen or listen but do not hear. Headlines of the following sort have become a commonplace: "All Too Often, The Doctor Isn't Listening, Studies Show," "Doctors Admit Ignoring Dying Patients' Wishes," "Failing to Discuss Dying Adds To Pain of Patient and Family."[17] But if doctors do not always listen, they also know what it is like not to feel free to be heard themselves or to discuss with others what they are doing. The first installment of a major three-part feature in the *Boston Globe* in 1993, titled "Death & the Doctor's hand," ran with a call-out prominently displayed just under the title: "Increasingly, secretly, physicians are helping the incurably ill to die."[18] Thus patients and doctors alike have reasons to wish for open discussions, which is one of the prime arguments Timothy Quill makes for legalizing physician-aid-in-dying. Doctors need to be able to consult with each other so they do not have to act privately and in secrecy when they are considering a patient's request for assistance in dying. Both doctor and patient will benefit, and so, in the end, will society as a whole.

The concern that allowing physicians to assist directly in the deaths of their patients would have a negative effect on the integrity of the medical profession—part of the so-called slippery-slope argument—has already been addressed. The specter is worth raising again, however, for it is regularly invoked by those who are opposed to legalizing physician-aid-in-dying. I said earlier that the chief problem with the argument was that it relied on an implicit empirical claim for which there is no possibility of any direct evidence until such assistance is legalized.

The issue is, however, more complicated than that, as James Rachels's discussion makes clear. In the first place, he insists that one version of the slippery-slope argument is a purely logical one (in other words, it is one that cannot be answered empirically). Only the second version of the argument, which is a psychological one, can be tested empirically. I argued that we cannot gather the evidence unless we legalize euthanasia. Rachels points out that even if we could show that there is a psychological possibility that some doctors will slide down just such a slippery slope, it does not follow that they all will. And the fact that some might, he says, is not sufficient reason for refusing to legalize euthanasia.[19] This seems to me right. We do not, for example, prohibit police officers from carrying guns or from being authorized to use them under certain circumstances simply because some police officers might slide down the slippery slope from permissible use to impermissible use—as we know some do.

Another argument sometimes proffered on behalf of maintaining proper standards for society goes like this: Some acts are simply so wrong that no one may be permitted to carry them out, not even those who do not believe they are wrong or harmful. This is the kind of argument often used by abortion foes, for instance: Abortion is murder, murder is a grave wrong, therefore abortion should be prohibited by law and anyone trying to procure or perform an abortion should be stopped. I have already mentioned the problems inherent in sectarian arguments.

A more thoroughgoing response to such arguments can be found in Judith Jarvis Thomson's *Realm of Rights* (1990). There she takes care to distinguish between two kinds of claims we have against others—one, "that they not cause us harm" ("The Harm Thesis") and two, "that they not cause us 'non–belief-mediated' distress" ("The Distress Thesis"). Both, however, are to be further distinguished from the desire we have that others not cause us distress that is "belief mediated." Harm and non–belief-mediated distress may both be caused by what Thomson calls

"trespass," which includes, for example, physical assault; the harm or distress caused in no way depends on anyone's beliefs. Belief-mediated distress, on the other hand (which involves feelings that can be either
rationally or irrationally held) is entirely dependent on the beliefs one
holds. If, for example, your beliefs are such that my walking ten feet in
front of you causes you distress, that is belief-mediated distress rather than
genuine harm. We do not have a claim against others that they not cause
us such distress (however good it might be that they not do so).[20]

The importance of this distinction cannot be overemphasized; it has
particularly dramatic application in both the abortion and the euthanasia debates. To take the abortion example mentioned above, briefly: The
fact that you *believe* abortion is murder does not *make* it murder. Thus although you are understandably distressed when you think about people
procuring or performing abortions, that distress is belief mediated—and
you have no claim against others that they not cause you such distress.
Though it might be a good thing if you were not caused such distress,that
is a separate matter.

Now take the example relevant here: You may *believe* that euthanasia,
or perhaps even any kind of physician-assisted death, is murder, but that
(again) is not enough to *make* it murder. Therefore, regardless of how distressed you are about euthanasia and other forms of physician-aid-in-
dying, you have no claims against others that they not cause you this
distress; your distress is wholly belief mediated. You may be quite genuinely outraged, or morally indignant, but your outrage and moral indignation are still outgrowths of your beliefs about euthanasia. As Thomson
rightly insists, "feelings of moral indignation"—notwithstanding their
force—"will not carry" the moral weight often placed on them. Thus the
most ardent and emotional, belief-mediated cries of distress in opposition
to physician-aid-in-dying can almost always be dismissed—not as unreal
but as morally irrelevant to the behavior of others.[21]

This is not at all to say there is no merit in the feelings or the beliefs
that people have. Rather, it is a reminder that *rational argument* must be
based on reasons that support a conclusion, not on emotional assertions
or sectarian beliefs. If those assertions and beliefs can be reformulated to
make them part of a sound argument, then debate over differences can
(and should) begin in earnest.

In point of fact, the more certain we are about our beliefs, the more likely
we are to become engaged in controversy. This can be a good thing. Controversy arises when we discover that others are equally "certain" about
a position diametrically opposed to our own. Such discoveries tend to
make us uncomfortable. But as philosopher Trudy Govier has argued,
controversy can "expose errors and omissions" as well as "assumptions
that have not been questioned," and it may help us "come to better
understand our own beliefs."[22] Such considerations are of paramount

importance; they may prove key to smoothing out the differences between Hospice and Hemlock. Thomson makes a similar point:

[W]hat the parties to a purely moral dispute try to do is to search for common moral ground: something that is in both their moral codes, that can be brought to bear on the issue in hand to settle it. That means that what X tries to do is to convict Y of failing to connect, either within Y's own moral code or across its boundary. It is because there is the possibility of success in doing this that one side can surprise the other and that one side can learn from the other, even if discovery of fact is not in question. Moreover, it is because there is the possibility of success in doing this that one side can be persuaded by the other and that moral arguments can be settled.[23]

By now it should be clear that there definitely *is* common ground between Hospice and Hemlock where precisely the kind of positive controversy Govier has in mind can be put to work, and where the possibility of success that Thomson heralds should give us hope. Our task should be to make sure the common ground is solid so that we can stand on it firmly. This will require capitalizing on shared sentiments, striving to understand the differences in beliefs, and using the controversy that is bound to arise—that already exists—in a constructive manner. In the end, the goal should be to bridge the gaps we cannot fill.

HEROIC COMPASSION: HOSPICE *AND* HEMLOCK

I said at the outset that I would focus my inquiry on what it is appropriate for dying persons to expect, desire, or request by way of assistance from their physicians and whether either Hospice or Hemlock alone can provide it. If we formulate the question with precision—Is true (and, yes, heroic) compassion to be found only through Hospice or only through Hemlock?—then I hope it has become obvious that the answer has to be a resounding "No." We cannot do justice to the complexity of the issue if we simply embrace the one and reject the other. When Hospice and Hemlock are under discussion, it cannot be a question of "or"; it has to be "both . . . and." (Recall Timothy Quill's insistence that he never talks about assisted dying without talking about hospice care, because it makes no sense to do otherwise.)

This position is also taken by a working party of the Institute of Medical Ethics (IME) in England. In a cautious statement on "assisted death" (reviewing the British Medical Association's euthanasia report of 1988), a heavy stress was put on the importance of pain relief: "Doctors hold relief of their patients' suffering to be their first and most rewarding duty." The report concludes with the following majority view:

A doctor, acting in good conscience, is ethically justified in assisting death *if the need to relieve intense and unceasing pain or distress caused by an incurable illness greatly outweighs the benefit to the patient of further prolonging his life.* . . . Assistance of death, however, is not justified *until the doctor and the clinical team are sure that the patient's pain and distress cannot be relieved by any other means—pharmacological, surgical, psychological, or social.*[24]

Here we see a very clear nod in the direction of Hemlock: A physician may under some circumstances be justified in assisting a patient's death. But Hospice also gets a strong endorsement for its characteristic emphasis on a team approach to care of the dying and the need to recognize that there are kinds of distress other than the purely somatic. (Not all Hospice supporters read the IME statement this way. Robert G. Twycross, failing to see the extent to which the statement extols and encourages Hospice policies, refers to the passage just quoted as a "utopian criterion" and goes on to insist that it "is time to remove the rose-tinted spectacles and to be realistic. The opportunity to opt out will probably *discourage* the patient and clinical staff from pursuing all other available avenues."[25] He gives no evidence for his claim.)

The Hemlock Society U.S.A. itself in a recent position statement makes a remarkably similar plea for melding what Hospice and Hemlock have to offer. Admiration is expressed for Hospice's "ability to provide compassionate care, to alleviate much of the suffering and pain of terminal illness, and to deal with the spiritual and psychological concerns of the patient and the family."[26] Yet some Hemlock supporters might also find the IME statement disappointing because it does not mention the rights involved. The endorsement of assisted death is limited to cases where pain relief has failed; thus it simply fails to address the questions raised by persons wanting to exercise a right to die for some other reason. The position statement of The Hemlock Society, not surprisingly, deals with this matter head on. Those patients whose pain cannot be relieved or who cannot (do not wish to) tolerate the side effects of whatever measures would be required to alleviate the pain, and those who cannot (do not wish to) tolerate the "indignity of the disease, the loss of control over bodily functions, the dependence and immobility," should not need "to make a choice between their autonomy to decide about the end of life and their ability to get high quality hospice care. Both options should be available." The statement then ends with two rhetorical questions and a direct statement about the need for both Hospice and Hemlock. "Why can't a person have a peaceful, gentle, quick and certain death in the presence of loved ones, even if they do not choose to live until the very last [possible] second? Why shouldn't people have this ultimate choice? It should not be Hemlock vs. Hospice but Hemlock *and* Hospice as options for a peaceful death."[27] This position is supported in at least some local

Hemlock chapters, as well, as evidenced by a letter to the editor from the chairman of the Greater Boston Hemlock Society, following a *Boston Globe* feature story on Hospice: "[Y]our portrayal of hospices as an alternative to physician-assisted suicide is off the mark. . . . [T]he two [are] compatible."[28]

Comfort care is extremely important, as Joanne Lynn (among others) has made vividly clear. We should all be able to agree on that. But *your* "comfort" cannot be allowed to stop just where *I* think it should, nor should *mine* end where *you* think it should. We may disagree, and then what is one to do? Comfort should extend as far as those in need of comfort think it should. And this is where the other question on which I said I would focus returns to center stage: What is it appropriate for the dying to expect, desire, or request by way of assistance from their physicians? I have hinted at fragmentary answers as I have gone along. It remains now to gather up the bits and pieces, to come to some kind of conclusion.

Throughout, I have assumed (as I said I would) that "compassionate" care is the goal of precisely the sort Hospice has endeavored to make commonplace. But if a large part of the point of Hospice's "caring to the end"[29] is to show respect not just for life but for the persons living those lives, it must also include respect for those persons' belief systems.

To be sure, there may be persons whose belief systems are completely at odds with basic morality. For that reason, "respect for . . . persons' belief systems" must come with a caveat. If a belief system allows arbitrary discrimination toward those who happen not to be liked—on grounds that have no moral significance (like hair or eye or skin color)—then we should work to see to it that discrimination based on such beliefs is outlawed. It becomes our job to point out the inherent unfairness and moral irrelevance of those beliefs. Ronald Dworkin, in his analysis of the 1996 Ninth and Second Circuit court decisions made absolutely clear that this was the key issue in those assisted-suicide cases. The "central question," he said, was this: "May a 'moral majority' limit the liberty of other citizens on no better ground than it disapproves of the personal choices they make?"[30] Judge Stephen Reinhardt of the Ninth Circuit answered that question in no uncertain terms:

Those who believe strongly that death must come without physician assistance are free to follow that creed, be they doctors or patients. They are not free, however, to force their views, their religious convictions, or their philosophies on all the other members of a democratic society, and to compel those whose values differ with theirs to die painful, protracted, and agonizing deaths.[31]

Thus we have to determine for ourselves just how to make autonomy, self-actualization, and choice—some of the important buzz-words among rights theorists—work for us. We have to decide for ourselves what "death with dignity" means for us personally. How important and difficult this is was being pointed out already twenty years ago. David L. Jackson and Stuart Youngner explored the ways in which too great a preoccupation with patient autonomy and the right to die with dignity "may lead physicians and patients to make clinically inappropriate decisions—precisely because sound clinical evaluation and judgment are suspended" out of deference to the patient's wishes.[32] A year earlier, another commentator had raised a related issue: "'Death with dignity' and 'a beautiful death' verge on becoming the new jargon of concern. But for whom are these expressions really meaningful? Do they describe the dying person's experience, or the observer's?"[33] Much more recently, another writer—attempting to separate the idea of "death with dignity" from euthanasia and assisted suicide—concluded that the phrase was "never very clear in the first place [and] should be given up."[34]

As we saw in the course of setting up model arguments, Hospice and Hemlock tend to view both "dignity" and "choice" rather differently. Hospice supporters are likely to say that human dignity is maintained by allowing people to make choices about how they will live life fully to the end. Hemlock supporters want to leave options open; they insist that, for some individuals, there may come a point in living life as fully as possible when dignity requires making the choice to die.

No one can possibly define generally or guess ahead of time when, in particular cases, such a point might come. Kirsten Backstrom, in a very thoughtful piece, reflects on her own experience with severe pain and debilitation. She stresses that opting too soon for assisted death could mean depriving oneself of life that could have considerable "quality" (and, presumably, dignity)—just not the kind of quality we think about when we are well. Yet she errs, it seems to me, in the reason she gives for thinking that assisted suicide is a danger. "I would like to know that I have the option of dying if pain becomes more than I can bear, but I wouldn't want to decide in advance how much I can bear," she writes.

"This is where . . . the danger of assisted suicide comes in."[35] And this is where she goes astray. Nothing about any rational proposal for making assisted suicide available would require persons to "decide in advance" how much pain they could bear. (A common misunderstanding about Living Wills and Health-Care Proxy statements is that one cannot change one's mind.)

A more likely scenario is one like that described by Sidney Wanzer, about his brother's decline and death from metastatic carcinoma of the lung. At his brother's request, Wanzer—a doctor—provided him with pills sufficient for him to end his own life. Dr. Wanzer also saw to it that his brother's pain medication was "upgraded drastically," so that "pain control was established." In the end, as Wanzer has recounted for numerous audiences, his "brother never used the pills, but they were a great comfort to him. He kept them immediately at hand in his bedside table and they clearly gave him a sense of control, which made all the difference in the world."[36] This, I submit, is the perfect paradigm for what a combined Hospice and Hemlock approach to dying would look like: Vigorous pain management (though it is all too typical, and sad, that the pain Wanzer's brother experienced apparently was not adequately managed until his brother the doctor arrived and became his advocate) coupled with an open option to choose death and the means to act on it "immediately at hand." Having the means (and thus the option) for an assisted death did not mean that Wanzer's brother had to "decide in advance" how much pain he could tolerate. Rather, it played a role in his ability to tolerate the pain (and perhaps loss of dignity) that he eventually experienced.

The issue of control, mentioned by Wanzer, raises a central question for any autonomous human being when it comes to questions of life and death: "Who is in charge?" Here, too, there is more than one way to look at it, as we have seen. Much of what Daniel Callahan says about the contemporary "quest for personal control [that] has . . . taken on an almost driven quality" is insightful; no doubt many of us *do* pursue control to excess. Yet it is clear that Callahan is expressing truths about himself that may not fit others, despite his attempt to generalize the point ("I have come to think that the preoccupation with control has become both subtly demeaning and socially troubling," he tells us.[37]). There is also Timothy Quill's reality, that the dying patient *should* be the one in control (to the extent possible). Your death should be your story, he told me, just as "my death is my story."[38]

Nonetheless, each of us is likely to need help telling our stories, bringing them to a satisfactory conclusion. Yet although explorations of the changing doctor-patient relationship purport to show we have made considerable progress, the continuing focus on that central dyad is misleading. Improvements in the way doctors deal with patients are real, to be sure; the authoritarian paternalism of yore is less in evidence today. But too much emphasis on doctor-patient interaction ignores the importance of other relationships in the dying person's life. We need to acknowledge that intimate and earnest talk between doctors and patients is not all that matters. Even when the doctor-patient discourse in a particular situation goes smoothly, and the communication seems effective, doctors and patients should not be the only actors. The dying need to be surrounded and uplifted by others. One of the great contributions of Hospice has been its emphasis on the need for a full-team approach, for the support of many people playing many different kinds of roles. Furthermore, learning how to die and how to care for the dying are part of an epic saga, a story that spills across generations.[39] Family, friends, clergy, neighbors may all appropriately encircle the dying person; communication takes many forms. Not all of them involve dialogue or even talk.

Of course we cannot all count on being fortunate enough to have such a full circle of persons to surround us as we approach death. Tolstoy's Ivan Ilyich lacked the desirable support in some important regards. But there was on hand a servant, a simple peasant boy, who knew how to *be* with a dying person. The lad raised the dying man's legs so they would not ache and rested them on his own shoulders, an act of communication that goes far beyond words and dialogue.[40] Just so, proponents of Hospice who focus much of their energy on developing a team to care for the dying person (and the family) also show a deep understanding that communication entails, among other things, surrounding an individual with support of whatever sort is needed. A contemporary Russian writer, Ludmila Ulitskaya, demonstrates an understanding of this important point in her book *The Funeral Party*. There the dying man's last days are filled with friends who both literally and figuratively lift him up.[41]

Assuring that we have a certain right does not, as we have seen, tell us what is the right thing to do. We will each still need to do our moral homework, so to speak. That will probably have to include sorting out the details of a relationship with our doctors, and it certainly needs to include putting into writing something of what we think appropriate for ourselves. Whether this written memorandum takes the form of a "living will" or is simply a statement of beliefs, dated and signed, is less important than that it be written down and that friends and family know where to find it. Choosing a health-care proxy to make our medical decisions for us if we become incapacitated and formally documenting that choice are critical steps. (A reminder of the importance came in a California Supreme Court decision in 2001 that sharply limited a family's right to have life support removed from a relative no longer competent to make his or her own decisions regarding medical treatments. The justices "emphasized the narrow scope of their ruling, saying it affected only cases involving patients who are conscious, who would die without life support, and who have not left formal directions for health care or legally appointed anyone to make such decisions should they ever be unable to make them." It is likely, however, to affect thousands of people.[42]) Then, too, our "homework" may need to include trying to trace our life's trajectory—however difficult and painful that might turn out to be. "These profound life-and-death issues and uncertainties are difficult to grasp, and many people would prefer to avoid them. Yet they do so at their peril," warns Timothy Quill.[43]

Facing these issues is important not least because part of what makes a particular end-of-life decision "good" or "appropriate" is that it fits the overall pattern of the dying person's life. Decisions about appropriateness will be made differently by different people—which is part of why it matters to have both Hospice and Hemlock available. Although many proponents of Hospice (chief among them Cicely Saunders herself) continue to take an unwavering stand in opposition to anything that might be called "Hemlock," there are cracks in the wall. Not only do we find former Hospice medical directors like Timothy Quill insisting on the need to make room for assisted dying along with greater availability of Hospice-like care; there are also occasional articles in Hospice journals urging a less doctrinaire approach to care for the dying. A Hospice nurse in California wrote (in 1994) that "Hospice tries hard, but we cannot guarantee every patient a peaceful death, and we know it. . . . Despite its rhetoric and good intentions, today's hospice care does not provide what many patients are genuinely seeking—a voice in the type of help they want."[44] (The contrast with Ira Byock's insistence that "[p]hysical suffering can *always* be alleviated"—a more typical Hospice line—is dramatic.[45])

Even more remarkable was the answer to a question about how physicians should respond to a request to "Help me die" that was given by Hospice doctor Joel Potash, in Syracuse. In a special report on "Doctors and Death" in the *New York Times* (in 1997), we are told that Potash "believes that a small number of terminally ill patients are justified in wanting to commit suicide and that doctors should be allowed to help."[46] Around the same time, a Hospice medical director in Canada wrote as follows: "Many people who have devoted their lives to the care of the dying are not opposed to physician-assisted suicide. Such people believe it should be available as one of several options, and, therefore, do not believe that promoting hospice and advocating for the availability of regulated physician-assisted suicide are contradictory goals." He ended his article with exactly the point I have tried to make: "When we fall to the extremes, we take choices away from those . . . we believe we are helping. But, there is a middle ground. When we aim for that middle ground, we all win."[47] Yet clearly there are still many who do not agree.[48]

Another aspect of the way in which Hospice and Hemlock not only do not have contradictory goals but actually share a message is described by sociologist Tony Walter. He points out that what he calls "the euthanasia lobby" and "the hospice lobby" (my "Hemlock" and "Hospice") are both concerned that physical death should not be separated by too great a time or distance from "social death." Both "are distressed by the sight of patients so wracked by pain or so ignored by hospital or nursing home that they would be (as we sometimes say) better off dead. Euthanasia would bring forward physical death so that it coincides with social death; good hospice care pushes back social death until the moment of physical death."[49]

Whether having "Hemlock" available requires legalizing physician-aid-in-dying is not so clear as one might hope it would be. My own position is that legalization should not be necessary, but that it probably would be a good thing if it were to take place. Chief among the reasons is that the burden of making a decision about when to die, in cases where one even has the opportunity, should be carried primarily by the dying person. (The story of my death should be my story, the story of your death should be your story.) Such decisions should not be turned into legal as well as moral burdens for the doctor. If physician assistance of the kind I have been talking about were legal, the likelihood that physician-aid-in-dying would be part of a carefully considered continuum of care where physicians had opportunities to consult freely and openly with colleagues (as Timothy Quill fervently urges they should) would be that much greater.

Explicitly legalized or not, however, the option needs to be open for doctors and patients together to decide what is most appropriate, most compassionate, in a particular situation. (A particularly affecting story of how one woman made choices about her own death with the encouragement of her doctor-son and the support of her own physician—she "relished her last piece of chocolate, and then stopped eating and drinking"—is told by David Eddy, at his late mother's request.[50]) It should be possible, as physician Lonny Shavelson has pointed out, to cross the divide between Hospice and Hemlock. It should be possible to make a leap from a

compassionate desire to offer the best of care to everyone who is dying, to a law that would incorporate the best of the philosophies of hospice and Hemlock. A system could be developed so that when any patient who is near death asks for assistance in suicide or for active euthanasia, a hospice physician and nurse are rapidly made available to evaluate the patient's care and to offer the patient and family the best of their skills. . . . [I]ntegral to this plan would be an understanding that, if as sometimes will happen, the best efforts of hospice to alleviate a patient's suffering fail, and firm and repeated requests to have help to die more quickly continue—then it is the patient's wish, not hospice philosophy, that is finally respected.[51]

The heroic compassion we are most of us searching for is, I am convinced, best expressed by *caring* all the way to the end, by offering comfort in myriad ways, and by physicians giving aid in dying—if that is called for.

NOTES

1. Simone de Beauvoir (Claude Francis and Fernande Goutier, trans.), *Who Shall Die?* (Florissant, Mo.: River Press, 1983) [*Les bouches inutiles* (Paris: Gallimard, 1945)], p. 61. I am indebted to Nancy Bauer for drawing this work to my attention.

2. Ray Monk, *Ludwig Wittgenstein: The Duty of Genius* (New York: Free Press, 1990), p. 579, quoting what Mrs. Joan Bevan—present at Wittgenstein's death—said were the philosopher's last words.

3. "Most Americans die in facilities, poll says," *BG* (11 Sept. 2000): A18. See also David Kessler, "A good, comfortable, pain-free ending," *BG* (24 Aug. 2001): A25.

4. Sharon Begley, "The Moment of Death," *Newsweek* (25 Nov. 1996): 65.

5. See Paul Wilkes, "Dying Well Is the Best Revenge," *NYT Mag.* (6 July 1997): 34, 38.

6. Ira Byock, *Dying Well: The Prospect for Growth at the End of Life* (New York: Riverhead Books, 1997), p. 57 (called by one Hospice executive director "the best recent book on death and dying"; Paul Montgomery, personal communication).

7. Anne Murphy (an internist), quoted in Wilkes, "Dying Well," *NYT Mag.*: 32.

8. Near the end of the play *Whose Life Is It Anyway?* the protagonist makes the point explicit: "The cruelty doesn't reside in saving someone or allowing them to die. It resides in the fact that the choice is removed from the man concerned." Brian Clark, *Whose Life Is It Anyway?* (New York: Avon Books, 1978), p. 141.

9. Ronald Dworkin, *Life's Dominion: An Argument About Abortion, Euthanasia, and Individual Freedom* (New York: Knopf, 1993), p. 117.

10. See Robert Pear, "More Patients in Hospice Care, But for Far Fewer Final Days," *NYT* (18 Sept. 2000): A23.

11. Sidney H. Wanzer, *The End of Life: How to Deal with the System, A Practical Guide for Patients and Families* (Denver, Colo.: The Hemlock Society, 2001), pp. 20–21.

12. For an account of a liberal society based on toleration of sectarian differences, see John Rawls, *Political Liberalism* (New York: Columbia University Press, 1993).

13. Daniel Callahan, *The Troubled Dream of Life: Living With Mortality* (New York: Simon & Schuster, 1993), pp. 20, 130–31, 132, 150, 153–55.

14. Peter Steinfels, "Beliefs: Doctor-assisted suicide in Oregon . . . ," *NYT* (7 Mar. 1998): A7.

15. Dworkin, *Dominion,* pp. 214, 215.

16. Dworkin, *Dominion,* p. 217.

17. Daniel Goleman, "All Too Often, The Doctor Isn't Listening, Studies Show," *NYT* (13 Nov. 1991): C1, C15; Jane E. Brody, "Doctors Admit Ignoring Dying Patients' Wishes," *NYT* (14 Jan. 1993): A18; and Esther B. Fein, "Failing To Discuss Dying Adds To Pain of Patient and Family," *NYT* (5 Mar. 1997): A21–22.

18. Dick Lehr, "Death & the Doctor's hand," *BG* (25 Apr. 1993): 1. See also by Lehr, "More learn of a practice long hidden," *BG* (26 Apr. 1993): 1, 8–9, and "Physicians face wrenching choices," *BG* (27 Apr. 1993): 1, 6–7.

19. James Rachels, *The End of Life: Euthanasia and Morality* (Oxford: Oxford University Press, 1986), pp. 172–75.

20. Judith Jarvis Thomson, *The Realm of Rights* (Cambridge, Mass.: Harvard University Press, 1990), pp. 250–253 and ff.

21. See Thomson, *Realm,* p. 257 and pp. 249–62 generally.

22. Trudy Govier, "Argument, Adversariality, and Controversy," in Frans van Eemeren, Rob Grootendorst, J. Anthony Blair, and Charles A. Willard, eds., *Proceedings of the Fourth ISSA Conference on Argumentation* (Amsterdam: Sic Sat, 1999), p. 263. The paper was reprinted in her *Philosophy of Argument* (Newport News, Va.: Vale Press, 1999).

23. Thomson, *Realm,* p. 27.

24. Institute of Medical Ethics Working Party on the Ethics of Prolonging Life and Assisting Death, "Assisted death," *Lancet* 336 (8 Sept. 1990): 613 (emphasis added).

25. Robert G. Twycross, "Assisted death: a reply," *Lancet* 336 (29 Sept. 1990): 797, 798.

26. Faye Girsh (Executive Director, Hemlock Society U.S.A.), "Hemlock and Hospice: A Position Statement" [8 June 1998].

27. Girsh, "Hemlock and Hospice" [1998].

28. Nancy S. Dorfman (letter to the editor), "When pain is too much," *BG* (30 June 1996): 68.

29. Cicely Saunders used the phrase as a title for one of her articles. See her "Caring to the end," *Nursing Mirror* (4 Sept. 1980): [no pg. nos.].

30. Ronald Dworkin, "Sex, Death, and the Courts," *The New York Review* (8 Aug. 1996): 44.

31. *Compassion in Dying v. Washington*, 79 F.3d 790, 839 (1996). The Hemlock Society was so taken with this ringing condemnation of the refusal to acknowledge a right to physician-assisted suicide that it had peel-off stickers made up with the quotation—but, as we know from the decisions that came down in June 1997, the Supreme Court did not agree with Judge Reinhardt. See *Washington v. Glucksberg*, 521 U.S. 702 (1997) and *Vacco v. Quill*, 521 U.S. 793 (1997).

32. David L. Jackson and Stuart Youngner, "Patient Autonomy and 'Death with Dignity,'" *NEJM* 301, no. 8 (23 Aug. 1979): 405.

33. Norman Klein, "Is There a Right Way to Die?" *Psychology Today* (Oct. 1978): 122.

34. Christopher Miles Coope, "Death with Dignity," *HCR* 27, no. 5 (Sept.-Oct. 1997): 38.

35. Kirsten Backstrom, "What Quality?" *Friends Journal* (Feb. 1999): 16. I am indebted to Craig Putnam for bringing this article to my attention.

36. Sidney H. Wanzer, "Risky and Nonrisky Acts," *Harvard Med. Alum. Bull.* (Winter 1997): 31.

37. Daniel Callahan, *The Troubled Dream of Life: Living with Mortality* (New York: Simon & Schuster, 1993), pp. 16, 17; see also pp. 153–55 and generally.

38. See the Profile of Quill in Ch. 4. For a powerful dialogue on the subject of control, see "Confronting Death: Who Chooses, Who Controls? A Dialogue between Dax Cowart and Robert Burt," *HCR* 28, no. 1 (Jan.-Feb 1998): 14–24.

39. This way of thinking about how end-of-life decision-making is (or should be) carried out was suggested by Steven H. Miles, personal communication.

40. Leo Tolstoy, *The Death of Ivan Ilyich and Other Stories* (New York: New American Library, 1960 [*The Death of Ivan Ilyich*, 1887]), pp. 136–138.

41. Ludmila Ulitskaya (Cathy Porter, trans.), *The Funeral Party* (New York: Schocken Books, 1999).

42. Evelyn Nieves, "California Justices Limit Families' Right to End Life Support," *NYT* (10 Aug. 2001): A10. See also Maura Dolan, "Calif. high court sets right-to-die standards," *BG* (10 Aug. 2001): A3.

43. Timothy E. Quill, *Death and Dignity: Making Choices and Taking Charge* (New York: Norton, 1993), p. 74.

44. Theresa M. Stephany, "Assisted suicide: How hospice fails," *Am. Jrnl. of Hospice & Palliative Care* (July/Aug. 1994): 5.

45. Byock, *Dying Well*, p. xiv (emphasis in the original).

46. Elizabeth Rosenthal, "When a Healer Is Asked, 'Help Me Die,'" *NYT* (13 Mar. 1997): A1.

47. John L. Miller, "Hospice care or assisted suicide: A false dichotomy," *Am. Jrnl. of Hospice & Palliative Care* (May/June 1997): 134.

48. Clive Seale, "Social and ethical aspects of euthanasia: a review," *Progress in Palliative Care* 5, no. 4 (1997): 143, cites to other examples where Hospice has been criticized or where it has been suggested that Hospice and Hemlock have "a unity of purpose" (and to the sometimes-outraged replies to these suggestions).

49. Tony Walter, *The Revival of Death* (London: Routledge, 1994), p. 51.

50. David Eddy, "A Conversation With My Mother," *JAMA* 272, no. 3 (20 July 1994): 181.

51. Lonny Shavelson, *A Chosen Death: The Dying Confront Assisted Suicide* (Berkeley: University of California Press, 1998 [New York: Simon & Schuster, 1995]), pp. 226–27.

For Further Reading

The books listed here constitute only a fraction of the vast literature available today on many different aspects of end-of-life decision-making. Most of these works were cited or quoted in this book. The "Notes" sections at the end of each chapter also provide references to articles in magazines, professional journals, and newspapers that are well worth reading. Some of the books listed in this chapter are genuine classics in the field of "death studies," while others are quite new. Several are scholarly, written by philosophers or physicians, while many (including some of those written by physicians) are much easier reading. A fair number have been on the best-seller list and will be easy to find. Others will require a bit more effort on the part of an interested reader. Each has much to recommend it.

The list of Web sites at the end of this chapter is also by no means a complete inventory of all that is available. It does, however, include resources on both sides of the Hemlock/Hospice divide. There is much to be learned by patient study of these sites, just as there is much to be learned from reading even a few of the books listed here.

Albom, Mitch. *Tuesdays with Morrie: An Old Man, Young Man, and Life's Greatest Lesson*. New York: Doubleday, 1997.

Ariès, Philippe. *The Hour of Our Death*. New York: Oxford University Press, 1991.

Battin, Margaret Pabst. *The Least Worst Death: Essays in Bioethics on the End of Life*. Oxford: Oxford University Press, 1994.

Beauchamp, Tom L., ed. *Intending Death: The Ethics of Assisted Suicide and Euthanasia*. Upper Saddle River, N.J.: Prentice Hall, 1996.

Becker, Ernest. *The Denial of Death*. New York: Free Press, 1973.

Brock, Dan W. *Life and Death: Philosophical Essays in Biomedical Ethics*. Cambridge: Cambridge University Press, 1993.

Byock, Ira. *Dying Well: The Prospect for Growth at the End of Life.* New York: Putnam/Riverhead Books, 1997.

Callahan, Daniel. *The Troubled Dream of Life: Living with Mortality.* New York: Simon & Schuster, 1993.

Devlin, Patrick. *Easing the Passing: The Trial of Dr. John Bodkin Adams.* London: Bodley Head, 1985.

Dworkin, Ronald. *Life's Dominion: An Argument About Abortion, Euthanasia, and Individual Freedom.* New York: Knopf, 1993.

Feifel, Herman, ed. *The Meaning of Death.* New York: McGraw-Hill, 1959.

Feldman, Fred. *Confrontations with the Reaper: A Philosophical Study of the Nature and Value of Death.* New York: Oxford University Press, 1992.

Gavin, William Joseph. *Cuttin' the Body Loose: Historical, Biological, and Personal Approaches to Death and Dying.* Philadelphia: Temple University Press, 1995.

Glaser, Barney G., and Anselm L. Strauss. *Awareness of Dying.* Chicago: Aldine, 1965.

Glick, Henry R. *The Right to Die: Policy Innovation & Its Consequences.* New York: Columbia University Press, 1992.

Gomez, Carlos. *Regulating Death: Euthanasia and the Case of the Netherlands.* New York: Free Press, 1991.

Griffiths, John, Alex Bood, and Heleen Weyers. *Euthanasia and Law in the Netherlands.* Amsterdam: Amsterdam University Press, 1998.

Groopman, Jerome. *The Measure of Our Days: New Beginnings at Life's End.* New York: Viking, 1997.

Hendin, Herbert. *Seduced by Death: Doctors, Patients and the Dutch Cure.* New York: Norton, 1997.

Humphry, Derek. *Final Exit: The Practicalities of Self-Deliverance and Assisted Suicide for the Dying.* Eugene, Ore.: The Hemlock Society, 1991.

Humphry, Derek, and Mary Clement. *Freedom to Die: People, Politics, and the Right-to-Die Movement.* New York: St. Martin's Press, 1998 [updated in 2000].

Keizer, Bert. *Dancing with Mister D: Notes on Life and Death.* New York: Talese/Doubleday, 1997.

Kevorkian, Jack. *Prescription: Medicide—The Goodness of Planned Death.* Buffalo, NY: Prometheus Books, 1991.

Kübler-Ross, Elisabeth. *On Death and Dying.* New York: Macmillan/Collier Books, 1993.

Lynn, Joanne, ed. *By No Extraordinary Means.* Bloomington: Indiana University Press, 1986.

Misbein, Robert I. *Euthanasia: The Good of the Patient, The Good of Society.* Frederick, Md.: University Publishing Group, 1992.

Mitford, Jessica. *The American Way of Death Revisited.* New York: Knopf, 1998.

Momeyer, Richard W. *Confronting Death.* Bloomington: Indiana University Press, 1988.

Mor, Vincent, David S. Greer, and Robert Kastenbaum, eds. *The Hospice Experiment.* Baltimore: Johns Hopkins University Press, 1988.

Munley, Anne. *The Hospice Alternative: A New Context for Death and Dying.* New York: Basic Books, 1983.

Nuland, Sherwin B. *How We Die: Reflections on Life's Final Chapter*. New York: Knopf, 1994.

Palmer, Greg. *Death: The Trip of a Lifetime*. New York: HarperSan Francisco, 1993.

Quill, Timothy E. *Death and Dignity: Making Choices and Taking Charge*. New York: Norton, 1993.

————. *A Midwife Through the Dying Process: Stories of Healing & Hard Choices at the End of Life*. Baltimore: Johns Hopkins University Press, 1996.

Rachels, James. *The End of Life: Euthanasia and Morality*. Oxford: Oxford University Press, 1986.

Saunders, Cicely, and Robert Dunlop. *Living with Dying: A Guide to Palliative Care*. Oxford: Oxford University Press, 3d ed., 1995.

Shavelson, Lonny. *A Chosen Death: The Dying Confront Assisted Suicide*. Berkeley: University of California Press, 1998.

Sheehan, Denice C., and Walter B. Forman, eds. *Hospice and Palliative Care: Concepts and Practice*. Sudbury, Mass.: Jones and Bartlett, 1996.

Siebold, Cathy. *The Hospice Movement: Easing Death's Pains*. New York: Twayne, 1992.

Spiro, Howard M., Mary G. McCrea Curnen, Enid Peschel, and Deborah St. James, eds. *Empathy and the Practice of Medicine*. New Haven, Conn.: Yale University Press, 1993.

Spiro, Howard M., Mary G. McCrea Curnen, and Lee Palmer Wandel, eds. *Facing Death: Where Culture, Religion, and Medicine Meet*. New Haven, Conn.: Yale University Press, 1996.

Stoddard, Sandol. *The Hospice Movement: A Better Way of Caring for the Dying*. New York: Vintage, 1992.

Thomson, Judith Jarvis. *The Realm of Rights*. Cambridge, Mass.: Harvard University Press, 1990.

Wanzer, Sidney H. *The End of Life: How to Deal with the System, A Practical Guide for Patients and Families*. Denver: The Hemlock Society, 2001.

Webb, Marilyn. *The Good Death: The New American Search to Reshape the End of Life*. New York: Bantam, 1996.

WEB SITES

American Academy of Hospice and Palliative Medicine. http://www.aahpm.org

American Board of Hospice and Palliative Medicine. http://www.abhpm.org

Americans for Better Care of the Dying. http://www.abcd-caring.org

Approaching Death: Improving Care at the End of Life. http://www.nap.edu/readingroom

Before I Die. http://www.wnet.org.bid.index.html

Dying Well [Ira Byock]. http://www.dyingwell.org

ERGO [Derek Humphry]. http://www.FinalExit.org/dhumphry

The Hemlock Society USA. http://www.hemlock.org

Last Acts [Coalition of many groups involved in end-of-life care]. http://www.lastacts.org

National Hospice and Palliative Care Organization. http://www.NHPCO.org

NPR. The End of Life: Exploring Death in America. http://www.NPR.org
Oregon Death with Dignity Center. http://www.dwd.org
Partnership for Caring. http://www.partnershipforcaring.org
PBS. On Our Own Terms: Moyers on Dying. http://www.pbs.org/onourownterms
Project on Death in America [Soros Foundation]. http://www.soros.org/
    death.html

Index

Abandonment, of patients by doctors, 2, 25, 138, 167
ABCD (Americans for Better Care of the Dying), 21 n.50, 37, 172
Abortion, 88, 183, 184
Academy of Hospice and Palliative Medicine, 33
Adams, John Bodkin, 147 n.147
Adkins, Janet, 106–7, 110, 112, 115, 132
Admiraal, Pieter: quoted, 102 n.80
AIDS, 12, 95–96
American College of Physicians, 110
American Medical Association (AMA), House of Delegates, statement of, quoted, 86
American Society of Internal Medicine, 89, 110
American Society on Aging, 54
American Euthanasia Society, 45
The American Way of Death (Mitford), 7–8
Angell, Marcia: quoted, 152–53
Annas, George: quoted, 50
Apollo, 26
Apology (Plato), 44
The Arc, 22 n.54, 43
Ariès, Philippe, 14; quoted, 4–5, 26
Asclepius, 26
Ashcroft, John, 78, 99 n.36, 121

Argument: best-interests, 154; for Assistance, 74, 77–82; from Autonomy, 73–74, 75–81, 163; from Law, 73, 74–77. *See also* Dignity-of-life argument; Slippery-slope argument; Pain argument; Substituted judgement
Assistance. *See* Argument, for Assistance
Australia, 38, 143 n.83
Autonomy: cluster-right to die, 77; futility prevails over, 16; importance of, for Hemlock, 51, 65–66, 92, 154, 155, 156, 179, 180; patient, 47, 138, 149, 150–51, 162, 180, 188–89, 190, 194 n.8; principle of, 73, 153, 154; source of claim-right to die, 77; source of immunity-right to die, 76; source of privilege-right to die, 76–77; source of power-right to die, 77. *See also* Argument, from autonomy; Self-determination
Awareness of Dying (Glaser and Strauss), 7

Backstrom, Kirsten: quoted, 189
Baines, Mary, 58 n.43, 98–99 n.25
Barber v. Superior Court, 98 n.11

Barnard, David: quoted, 87
Baron, Charles: quoted, 151
Bartling v. Superior Court, 98 n.11
"Bathtub example." *See* Rachels, James,
    "Bathtub example"
Battin, Margaret Pabst, 125, 131; quoted,
    49, 124, 128
Beardsley, Elizabeth: quoted, 150
Beauchamp, Thomas, 86–87, 157
Becker, Ernest, 6, 7, 8; quoted, 5
Belgium, 144 n.105
Belief-mediated distress, 76, 185. *See
    also* "The Distress Thesis"
Beneficence: principle of, 16, 151, 152,
    154, 162, 173 n.16; Hospice view of,
    154
Berger, Jean: quoted, 27
Best-interests, patient's, 151. *See also*
    Argument, best-interests
Bok, Sissela, 91
Bood, Alex. *See* Griffiths, John, Alex
    Bood, and Heleen Weyers
Bouvia, Elizabeth, 67, 98 n.24
Bouvia v. Superior Court, 67, 98 n.24
Brewer, Colin, 60 n.89; quoted, 60 n.90,
    99 n.35
British Medical Association (BMA),
    1988 report on euthanasia, 186
Brock, Dan W.: quoted, 87, 157
Brody, Baruch: quoted, 87
Brody, Howard: quoted, 47
Burials, 7
Byock, Ira: quoted, 33, 179, 192

California, 2, 17 n.5, 103 n.91, 118,
    191, 194; *Superior Court*, 67
Callahan, Daniel, 5, 8, 182; quoted, 14,
    127–28, 133, 189, 190
Canada, 192
Canterbury v. Spence, 67
Caplan, Arthur: quoted, 50
Cardiopulmonary resuscitation (CPR),
    16, 38
Cardozo, Benjamin: quoted, 67
"Care of strangers," 30
Caring vs. curing, 4, 27, 35, 133, 167
Catholic Church, opposition to
    legalization of euthanasia, 118, 119

Center for Bioethics (Univ. of Minnesota),
    120
Center for Ethics and Humanities in
    the Life Sciences (Michigan State
    Univ.), 47
Center for Ethics in Healthcare
    (Oregon Health Sciences Univ.), 121
Center for the Evaluative Clinical
    Sciences (Dartmouth Medical
    School), 170
The Center to Improve Care of the
    Dying (George Washington Univ.),
    21 n.50, 37, 172
Choice in Dying, 45
*A Chosen Death: The Dying Confront
    Assisted Suicide* (Shavelson), 111
Christians, 30
Claims, 70. *See also under particular
    rights*
Clement, Mary, 53
Cluster-rights, 70, 75, 77, 81, 162
Cobbs v. Grant: quoted, 67
Cohen, Herbert, 126; contrast with
    Kevorkian, 131; profile of (and
    quoted), 129–32; view of Hospice,
    130
"Comfort care," 31, 166–67, 188
Compassion, 2, 3, 15, 17, 18 nn.9, 11,
    16, 28, 29, 33, 39, 48, 168; heroic, 3,
    186–93
Compassion in Dying (Washington), 45
Conant, Loring: quoted, 89
Concern for Dying, 45
Connecticut, 38
Consent, informed, 66–67, 75, 150
Cooper, Megan McAndrew: quoted, 166
Costs, health-care, 1, 43
CPR. *See* Cardiopulmonary
    resuscitation
Crito (Plato), 91
Cruzan, Nancy, 45
*Cruzan v. Director, Missouri
    Department of Health*, 45, 49, 61 nn.
    101, 102

Dach, Simon: quoted, 149
*Dancing with Mister D: Notes on Life
    and Death* (Keizer), 8, 131

Daniels, Norman, 100 n.42, 153
de Beauvoir, Simone: quoted, 177
Death: as a harm, 27; as event, 14; as
    evil, 4, 5; as lonely experience, 6; as
    ritual, 26; as taboo, 1, 6, 17 n.2;
    attitudes toward, 26; causes of, 26;
    constructing the concept of, 39;
    definition of, 11, 13, 14; denial of, 7,
    170; fear of, 5, 7; foreseen but not
    intended, 89, 90 (*see also* Doctrine of
    double effect); "hidden," 26;
    "social," 22 n.64; "tame," 14, 26;
    "trajectories of," 170; "wild," 14. *See
    also* Dying
*Death and Dignity: Making Choices and
    Taking Charge* (Quill) "Death
    awareness" movement, 8
Death studies. *See* Thanatology
"Death with dignity," 188–89
Death with Dignity Act, Oregon
    (ODDA), 17 n.5, 46, 55, 78, 118–19,
    119–20, 121, 142 n.78, 143 n.86
"Debbie," 106, 107, 108–9, 110, 118, 132
Decision-making, 170; shared, 165, 175
    n.35
Decision(s), end-of-life, 16, 133, 134,
    137, 138, 180, 189–90, 191–92
Devlin, Patrick, 147 n.147
The Denial of Death (Becker), 5, 6
Diane, 106, 108–10, 111, 114, 136, 165
Dignity-of-life argument, 160–61, 161
Disease, indignity of, 187
"The Distress Thesis," 184
DNR. *See* "Do Not Resuscitate" (DNR)
    order(s)
"Do Not Resuscitate" order(s), 16, 81
Doctors and death, history of, 25, 26
Doctor-patient dialogue, 164–68, 190.
    See also Quill, Timothy E., profile of
    (and quoted)
Doctor-patient relationship, 1, 27, 28,
    113, 114, 127, 132–35, 165
*Doctor Assisted Suicide and the
    Euthanasia Movement* (McCuen), 116
Doctrine of double effect, 88–93; in
    Catholic moral theology, 88;
    Hospice reliance on, 89; Quill's
    view of, 137

Doing Evil to Achieve Good (McCormick
    and Ramsey, eds.), 91
Drug Enforcement Administration, 121
Dutch Medical Association, 130
Duty of non-interference, 77
Duty to assist dying patient(s), 79–80
"Duty to die," 22 n.54. *See also*
    Saunders, Cicely, on "duty to die"
Dworkin, Ronald, 118; quoted, 11, 94,
    95, 96, 97, 122, 181, 182, 183, 188
Dying: as a benefit for patient, 151; as
    process, 14, 26, 45, 164; control over
    by patients, 36, 133, 138, 180 (*see
    also* Decision(s), end-of-life); fear of,
    4, 5, 7, 14; five stages of, 7, 20 n.38;
    loneliness of, 6; personal experience
    of, 179; "work" of, 179. *See also*
    Death
Dying, Death, and Bereavement (Corless,
    Germino, and Pittman, eds.), 8
Dying Well (Byock), 33

Eddy, David, 193
Egan, Timothy: quoted, 59
*The End of Life: How to Deal with the
    System, A Practical Guide for Patients
    and Families* (Wanzer), 1
England, 38, 41, 43; influence of Hospice
    in, 43
Epicurus: quoted, 5
"ERGO." *See* Euthanasia Research &
    Guidance Organization
"Euthanasia," broad meaning of, 167
Euthanasia, 12, 13, 49; active vs.
    passive, 42, 82, 90, 91; definition of,
    42, 93; difficulty in performing, 102
    n.80, 130; Hemlock support of, 83;
    Hospice opposition to, 83;
    legalization of, 42, 95–96, 118–29,
    184; non-voluntary vs. involuntary,
    127, 128; rational argument over,
    185; voluntary vs. involuntary, 42–
    43, 45, 83. *See also* The Netherlands,
    euthanasia in; Australia; Belgium
Euthanasia Educational Council, 61
    n.103
Euthanasia & Law in the Netherlands
    (Griffiths, Bood, and Weyers), 123

Euthanasia Research & Guidance
    Organization (ERGO), 46, 55
Euthanasia Society, 61 n.103
Evil. *See* Death, as evil

"Fair equality of opportunity." *See*
    Opportunity, fair equality of
"Fatal draught," prohibition of. *See*
    Hippocratic Oath, prohibition of
    fatal draught
Feifel, Herman, 6
Feldman, Fred, 5; quoted, 14
Fieger, Geoffrey, 117
Final Exit (Humphry), 43, 49, 50, 55,
    62 n.119
Fletcher, Joseph, 54; quoted, 94
Foley, Kathleen, 38; quoted, 37
Foot, Philippa: quoted, 88, 89
A Fortunate Man (Berger), 27
Frankl, Viktor: quoted, 61 n.94
Freedom to Die (Humphry and Clement),
    53
The Funeral Party (Ulitskaya), 191
Funerals, 7–8; cost of, 18 n.7
Futility, medical, 9, 13, 16–17, 23 n.71,
    151; prevails over autonomy, 16
Futility, other kinds of, 16–17

Gabriel, Trip: quoted, 53
Galen, 56 n.15
Ganzini, Linda, 120
gedogen, 124
Glaser, Barney, 6–7, 8
Gomez, Carlos, 125
The Good Death (Webb), 116, 171
"Good death" experience, 40
"Good death" movement, 45
Good Samaritan, 93
Goodman, Ellen, 124; quoted, 123
Govier, Trudy: quoted, 185
Greater Boston Hemlock Society, 188
Greece, ancient, 26
Griffiths, John. *See* Griffiths, John,
    Alex Bood, and Heleen Weyers
Griffiths, John, Alex Bood, and
    Heleen Weyers, 126, 131; quoted,
    23–24, 125, 126

"The Harm Thesis," 184
Harmon, Henry (Bud), 15
The Hastings Center, 149–50, 162
Hayward, John Stearns: quoted, 1
Health-care system, just, 153
Health Maintenance Organizations
    (HMOs), 134, 165
Helme, Tim: quoted, 89
"Hemlock": 44–51; agenda of, 45–46;
    broad meaning of term, 4, 11, 12,
    48; downside of, 50–51; history of,
    25; (internal) principles of, 159
Hemlock and Hospice. *See* Hospice,
    contrasted with Hemlock; Hospice
    and Hemlock
Hemlock (*conium maculatum*), 4, 18–19
    n.17, 44
Hemlock Society U.S.A., 45–48, 118,
    187; founding of, 44; 1993 mission
    statement, quoted, 46; 1998 position
    statement, quoted, 187
Hendin, Herbert, 129; quoted, 125,
    126
Herbert, Bob: quoted, 134
Hippocrates, 27, 28
Hippocratic Corpus, 28
Hippocratic Oath, 56 n.12; prohibition
    of "fatal draught" in, 28–30
Hohfeld, Wesley Newcomb, 69
Holland. *See* The Netherlands
"Hospice," broad meaning of term, 4,
    48; connotation of, 39; etymology
    of, 30
Hospice, contrasted with Hemlock,
    12, 17, 21–22 n.54, 47–48, 70–71, 82,
    88, 91–92, 149–61 passim
The Hospice Alternative (Munley), 34
Hospice and Hemlock: common
    ground of, 51, 65, 158, 178–83, 186,
    192; compatibility of, 48, 187–88;
    paradigm of joint approach, 189.
    See also Hospice, contrasted with
    Hemlock
Hospice and Hemlock (Hemlock
    Society), 44, 47, 48
Hospice and Palliative Care
    Medicine, 38

Hospice care, 11–12, 30–41, 58 nn.43, 45; availability of, 37–38, 39; importance of, 136

Hospice care vs. hospital care, 40

Hospice Federation of Massachusetts, 72

Hospice movement, modern, 11–12, 25, 31, 32–33; political nature of, 36

The Hospice Movement: A Better Way of Caring for the Dying (Stoddard), 34

Hospice organization, modern, 32, 39; Christian foundation of, 31–32, 42, 156, 180; current number of units in U.S.A., 59 n.70; downside of, 39–41; first unit in U.S.A., 37; ideology of, 21 n.52, 33–34, 41, 153; importance of palliative care for, 12, 34, 35, 59 n.72, 155, 156, 181; (internal) principles of, 158–59; media interest in, 11; variation in practices, 136–37, 192

Hospice services: controversy over, 35, 60 n.85, 58 n.55; public ignorance of, 21 n.49; public perception of, 59 n.71

Hospices, later history of, 31–32; origins of, 30

Hospitals, origins of, 30; conversion to hospices, 31

House of Lords Select Committee on Medical Ethics (England), 42, 60 nn.89, 90

How We Die: Reflections on Life's Final Chapter (Nuland), 8

Humphry, Derek, 43, 49–50, 127, 154; comment on Kevorkian, 54, 117–18; profile of (and quoted), 51–55; quoted, 46–47, 111

Immunities, 70. *See also under particular rights*

Incompetence, of dying patients, 13

India, ancient, 30

Informed consent. *See* Consent, informed

Institute for Healthcare Improvement, 21 n.50

Institute for the Study of Applied and Professional Ethics (Dartmouth College), 170

Institute of Medical Ethics (IME) (England), 186; statement of, quoted, 187

Integrity of the medical profession, 9, 93–97, 103 n.91, 109, 114, 155, 156, 163, 173 n.16; principle of, 152, 154–55, 162

Intention. *See* Doctrine of double effect

Ireland, 31

Jackson, David L.: quoted, 189

James, Henry, 15

Jecker, Nancy: quoted, 16

Joint Commission on Accreditation of Healthcare Organizations, 34

Just Health Care (Daniels), 153

Justice as fairness, principle of, 153, 155. *See also* Health-care system, just

Kaplan, Abraham: quoted, 157

Keizer, Bert, 8; as "wise clown," 131

Kendal at Hanover (N.H.), 170

Keown, John, 125

Kevorkian, Jack, 10, 11, 12, 22 n.54, 47, 51, 79, 93, 102 n.82, 107, 132, 158; attitude toward medical experiments on death row prisoners, 115; criminal conviction, 140 n.31; criticism, 113–15; influence of, on right-to-die debate, 46, 54–55, 140 n.29; in the media, 46, 51, 106, 112, 114, 117; profile of (and quoted), 115–18; support for, 110–11, 112–13. *See also* "Mercitron"; "Suicide machine"

Killing vs. letting die, 82–93, 126, 133; Hemlock view of, 91, 102 n.82; Hospice view of, 90; moral significance of distinction, 84, 86, 88

Knights Hospitaller of the Order of St. John, 30

Knowledge, medical: inherent uncertainty of, 20 n.46, 166

Koop, C. Everett: quoted, 113

Kübler-Ross, Elisabeth, 7, 8, 131

Law. *See* Argument, from Law
Lee, Barbara Coombs, 45
Lessenberry, Jack: quoted, 112
Levertov, Denise: quoted, 105
Liberty interest, 75
Life, quality of, 9, 31, 189; respect for
    human, 182, 189; sanctity of, 73, 164,
    182–83; trajectory of, 15, 161, 165
Living wills, 62 n.105, 189, 191
Lucretius: quoted, 5
Lundberg, George: quoted, 108
Lynn, Joanne, 18 n.7, 38, 188; profile
    of (and quoted), 168–72; quoted, 5,
    33, 34, 35, 36–37; view of Hospice,
    172

Maguire, Daniel: quoted, 164
Maine, 17 n.5
Malpractice, effect of fear of, 43, 178
Mandel, Tom, 106
Man's Search for Meaning (Frankl), 61
    n.94
Massachusetts, 45, 142 n.78; suicides
    inspired by *Final Exit* in, 50
The Meaning of Death (Feifel), 6
Measures, heroic, 38
Medical profession, integrity of the.
    See Integrity of the medical
    profession
Medical intervention, ordinary vs.
    extraordinary, 61 n.103, 86, 166
Medicare, 21 n.50, 36, 38, 171
"Medicaring," 21 n.50
"Mercitron," 107, 112, 113, 114. *See
    also* "Suicide machine"
"Mercy killing," 82, 116, 118
Merian's Friends Committee (Michigan),
    45
Mero, Ralph, 45
Michigan, 45, 111
A Midwife Through the Dying Process
    (Quill), 134, 135
Miller, Bruce, 150, 151
Mitford, Jessica, 7–8, 8
Momeyer, Richard: quoted, 91, 163
Moore, Francis: quoted, 135, 167

Moore, Merrill: quoted, 25
Morals and Medicine (Fletcher), 54
Morphine, use in pain relief, 58 n.43,
    89; killing with, 102 n.80, 107
Moslems, 30
Munley, Anne, 34; quoted, 40
Murphy, Donald: quoted, 151

National Council for Hospice and
    Specialist Palliative Care Services
    (England), 21 n.53
National Council of Hospice
    Professionals, 59 n.70
National Hospice and Palliative Care
    Organization (NHPCO), 12, 21 n.50,
    33, 34, 72
National Hospice Organization (NHO),
    12, 21 n.50, 32–33
Nazi eugenics, 45, 95
Nazis, use of euthanasia by, 45
The Netherlands, euthanasia in, 8, 10,
    20 n.37, 25, 96, 118, 122–29; Cicely
    Saunders, view of, 42. *See also*
    Cohen, Herbert, profile of (and
    quoted)
New York, 45, 122
Non-maleficence, principle of, 173 n.16
"Normal opportunity range," 153, 174
    n.21
Not Dead Yet, 22 n.54, 43
Nuland, Sherwin: quoted, 8
Nutrition, withdrawal of, 87

ODDA. *See* Death with Dignity Act,
    Oregon
On Death and Dying (Kübler-Ross), 7
Open Society Institute. *See* Project on
    Death in America
Opportunity, fair equality of, 153. *See
    also* "Normal opportunity range"
Oregon, 10, 45, 52, 106, 118–22, 138.
    See also Death with Dignity Act,
    Oregon
Oregon Health Sciences University
    (OHSU), 120, 121, 122
Organ transplant, 11
Oski, Frank: quoted, 112
Oliver, John, 43; quoted, 52

Our Bodies, Ourselves (Boston Women's Health Book Collective), 66

Pain: duty to relieve, 94; relief from, 44, 58 n.43, 65, 89, 186–87. *See also* Palliative care
Pain argument, 159–60, 160–61
Pain control, 35, 38, 40, 51, 178–79. *See also* Palliative care
Palliative care, 31, 43, 65, 131,168, 172, 178–79. *See also*, Hospice organization, modern, importance of palliative care for
Palmer, Greg: quoted, 35
Partnership for Caring, 45
PAS. *See* Physician-assisted suicide
Paternalism, 16, 150, 151, 153, 180, 190
Patients, vulnerable, 13, 22 n.56, 42, 119
Patients, welfare of. *See* Beneficence, principle of
Pence, Greg: quoted, 112
Perlin, Seymour, 157
Physician-aid-in-dying, 12–13, 13, 93–94, 102 n.82, 107–10, 114, 138, 163, 182, 183; legalization of, 118–29, 192–93; professional support for, 110
Physician-assisted suicide, 1, 10, 11, 12–13, 13, 49, 63 n.128; legalization of, 10, 110, 134, 142 n.78, 143 n.83; opposition to, 42, 172. *See also, e.g.,* Callahan, Daniel; Conant, Loring; Gomez, Carlos; Hendin, Herbert; Saunders, Cicely
Physician Orders for Life-Sustaining Treatment (POLST), 121–22
Physicians for Mercy, 112
Physicians for Compassionate Care, 121
Plato, 19 n.17
Potash, Joel, 192
Powers, 69–70. *See also under particular rights*
Prescription: Medicide (Kevorkian), 50, 106, 115
Pretty, Diane, 174 n.26
Pridonoff, John A.: quoted, 48

Priests, role of with the dying, 25
Primum non nocere, 27, 28, 56 n.12
Principle(s): clash of, 180; sectarian, 180–81. *See also* Autonomy, principle of; Beneficence, principle of; "Hemlock," (internal) principles of; Hospice organization, (internal) principles of; Integrity of the medical profession, principle of; Justice as fairness, principle of; Non-maleficence, principle of
Principles for evaluation: external, 149–57; internal, 157–61
Privacy, right to, 75
Privileges, 69. *See also under particular rights*
Project on Death in America, 38–39, 120
Proxy statement, health-care, 189, 191
Psychoanalysis, 6
PVS (persistent vegetative state), 151

Quill, Timothy E., 109–10, 111, 113, 114, 126, 133, 165, 190, 193; NEMJ article by, 106, 108–9, 116; comments on Kevorkian, 112, 117; contrast with Kevorkian, 135, 136; profile of (and quoted), 135–38; quoted, 40, 109, 110, 112, 120–21, 122, 152, 156, 163, 167, 183, 184, 191; view of Hospice, 136–37, 186
Quinlan, Karen Ann, 45, 61 n.102; *In re Quinlan*, 45, 49, 61 nn.101, 102, 67

Rachels, James, 85–86, 87, 184; "Bathtub example," 85, 89; quoted, 84
RADAR (England, disability charity), 22 n.54
Rawls, John, 153; quoted, 157
The Realm of Rights (Thomson), 67, 184
Regulating Death: Euthanasia and the Case of the Netherlands (Gomez), 125
Reilly, Thomas, 50
Reinhardt, Stephen, 195 n.31; quoted, 188
Religion, meaning of death in, 13, 15
Religious beliefs, 100 n.48, 162; argument based on, 164; as motivation for C. Saunders, 42

Remmelink Commission, 124, 127
Reno, Janet, 121
"Right" as noun vs. "right" as adjective, 68
Right to assistance in dying: as claim, 78, 79–80; as cluster, 77; as immunity, 78; as power, 78–79; as privilege, 78; Hemlock view of, 92–93
"Right to die," 4, 11, 12, 43, 67, 70–82, 98 n.24, 99 n.26; arguments for, 73–82; as claim, 77, 168; as cluster, 77; as immunity, 76, 77; as power, 75–76, 77; as privilege, 76–77; as ultimate civil liberty, 54, 154; denial of, 72; different senses of, 71, 189; Hemlock view of, 46, 73; Hospice view of, 72; meaning of, 80; Movement, 4, 61 n.103, 123
Right to life, 71, 100 n.40
Right to refuse treatment, 9, 67, 72, 73, 74, 77, 75, 81, 98 n.12, 150, 166; as claim, 75; as cluster, 75; as immunity, 75; as power, 74; as privilege, 75, 77
Rights: kinds of, 69–70; patient's, 1, 2; personal, 66, 67; strict, 69; significance of for morality, 68
"Rights revolution," 97 n.3
Rollin, Betty: quoted, 112
Rome, ancient, 5
Rothman, David: quoted, 67

Salgo v. Leland Stanford, Jr., University Board of Trustees, 67
"Sanctity of life," meaning of, 96. *See also* Life, sanctity of
Saunders, Cicely, 36, 38, 44, 83, 84, 167; as founder of modern Hospice movement, 31–32; on "duty to die," 43, 60–61 n.91, 71, 98–99 n.25; profile of (and quoted), 41–44; quoted, 32, 33, 35, 167; view of Hemlock, 42, 43, 192; view of Humphry, 43, 49, 55
Saunders, John: quoted, 16
Schloendorff v. Society of New York Hospital, 66
Schwartz, Morris, 105, 106

Seduced by Death: Doctors, Patients and the Dutch Cure (Hendin), 126
"Self-deliverance," 52, 63 n.128
Self-determination, right to, 46, 51, 163. *See also* Autonomy
Shakespeare, William: quoted, 65
Shavelson, Lonny, 2, 111; quoted, 62 n.119, 193
Sheffey, Lynn: quoted, 103 n.91
Shribman, David: quoted, 39
Siebold, Cathy, 36
Siegler, Mark, 150; quoted, 87
Slippery-slope argument, 94–95, 96, 103 nn.87, 90, 184
Snyder, Kristina: quoted, 49
Society for the Right to Die, 45, 61 n.103
Socrates, 18–19 n.17, 44, 91
Sovereign Foundation, 112
St. Christopher's Hospice (Sydenham), 32, 36, 40, 41, 43, 58 n.43, 136
Steinbock, Bonnie: quoted, 86
Steinfels, Peter: quoted, 182
St. Joseph's (London), 31, 32
St. Luke's House of the Dying Poor (Bayswater), 31, 32
Stoddard, Sandol, 34, 41–42
Strauss, Anselm, 6–7, 8
"Suicide machine," 10, 50, 110, 111. *See also* "Mercitron"
Suicide, 12, 53, 181; as equivalent to voluntary euthanasia, 99 n.35, 131; law on, 9–10; 109; importance of personal views on, 162; "rational," 44, 61 n.94; right to commit, 48–49, 75, 76, 77, 80
Sullivan, Thomas: quoted, 86
Substituted judgment, 151, 154. *See also* Argument, best-interests
SUPPORT, 165, 171
Supreme Court, United States, 45, 75, 122, 123, 135, 195 n.31

Tasma, David, 32
"Technological brinkmanship," 133
"Technological imperative," 27, 133
Technology, medical, 1, 9, 17 n.4, 25, 38, 39, 132. *See also* "Technological imperative"

Terminal illness, 12, 36, 46, 48, 171
Thomson, Judith Jarvis, 69, 87; quoted, 67, 70, 75, 76, 100 n.40, 184–85, 185, 186
Thanatology, 6, 10, 12, 19 n.30
The Tibetan Book of the Dead, 8, 20 n.43
Tolle, Susan: quoted, 121
Tolstoy, Leo, 191
Trespass, infringing claims by, 75, 184
Tribe, Laurence: quoted, 135
The Troubled Dream of Life: Living with Mortality (Callahan), 5, 182
Tucker Foundation (Dartmouth College), 170
Twycross, Robert: quoted, 187

Ulitskaya, Ludmila, 191
United States, hospice units in, 59 n.70; influence of Hospice in, 43; Senate Special Committee on Aging, 45. *See also* Supreme Court, United States

Vacco v. Quill, 17 n.6, 33, 122, 123, 135, 195 n.31
Values, diversity of, 137, 181
Vatican, declaration on euthanasia, 61 n.103
Voltaire: quoted, 19 n.33
Voluntary Euthanasia Society (VES) (England), 43, 45, 52

Wal, Gerrit van der, 127; quoted, 124, 126–27
Wallace, Mike, 117
Walter, Tony: quoted, 36, 192
Wanzer, Sidney, 2, 108, 181; quoted, 1–2, 3, 189–90
Washburn, Bradford: quoted, 112–13
Washington, 17 n.5, 45, 118, 122
Washington, D.C., 45
Washington v. Glucksberg, 17 n.6, 33, 122, 123, 195 n.31
Webb, Marilyn, 116; quoted, 171
Weisbard, Alan: quoted, 87
Weyers, Heleen. *See* Griffiths, John, Alex Bood, and Heleen Weyers
What Kind of Life? (Callahan), 133
Whose Life Is It Anyway? (Clark), 194 n.8
Wickett, Ann, 53
"Willing provider," 78, 79–80
Wings of the Dove (James), 15
Winkler, Earl: quoted, 82
Wittgenstein, Ludwig: quoted, 177
Woolfrey, Joan, 121
World Federation of Right to Die Societies, 10th International Conference of, 51–52, 52, 131

Youk, Thomas, 79, 102 n.82, 114, 117, 118
Youngner, Stuart: quoted, 16, 151, 189

About the Author

CONSTANCE E. PUTNAM is an independent scholar and writer who specializes in medical history and medical ethics. She lives in Concord, Massachusetts.